MW01490699

Presented to:

_____

From:

_____

For I know the plans I have for you…….(Jeremiah 29:11)

NEW BREAST FRIENDS

Surviving Cancer... Twice.

Diane Casperson with Cynthia Wakefield

WestBow
PRESS
A DIVISION OF THOMAS NELSON

Copyright © 2011 Diane Casperson with Cynthia Wakefield

All rights reserved. No part of this book may be used or reproduced by
any means, graphic, electronic, or mechanical, including photocopying,
recording, taping or by any information storage retrieval system
without the written permission of the publisher except in the case
of brief quotations embodied in critical articles and reviews.

WestBow Press books may be ordered through booksellers or by contacting:

WestBow Press
A Division of Thomas Nelson
1663 Liberty Drive
Bloomington, IN 47403
www.westbowpress.com
1-(866) 928-1240

Because of the dynamic nature of the Internet, any web addresses or
links contained in this book may have changed since publication and
may no longer be valid. The views expressed in this work are solely those
of the author and do not necessarily reflect the views of the publisher,
and the publisher hereby disclaims any responsibility for them.

Certain stock imagery © Thinkstock.
Any people depicted in stock imagery provided by Thinkstock are
models, and such images are being used for illustrative purposes only.

Scripture taken from the Holy Bible, New International Version®.
Copyright © 1973, 1978, 1984 Biblica.
Used by permission of Zondervan. All rights reserved.

ISBN: 978-1-4497-2214-2 (e)
ISBN: 978-1-4497-2216-6 (sc)
ISBN: 978-1-4497-2217-3 (hc)

Library of Congress Control Number: 2011913403

Printed in the United States of America

WestBow Press rev. date: 8/29/2011

DEDICATION

To my loving husband and children,

who I have been so graciously blessed with.

FOREWORD

By Diane Derheim
my treasured friend

I Heard the phone ringing in the midst of my quiet, peaceful day. The next sound was the compassion-filled voice of my husband saying, "You need to come to the hospital. Diane has cancer."

I Felt my knees weaken as my heart hurt, knowing that my friend's life would change as she knew it.

I Watched a young woman go into battle. The enemy's attack was quick and powerful as it reared its ugly head. Diane entered into her battle fighting with determination, grace, and dignity. She put faith in her God, embraced the strength of her loving family and friends, and formed a plan of attack. This was an all-out war against cancer. As she aggressively fought this battle, she discovered strength and comfort within the encouragement of her army of supporters. I saw the struggles and the tears, and I witnessed the battle scars of this warrior. I saw the relentless attacks, causing her to return into the hostile battle with even more rigor and determination. As the events of the battles unfolded, I watched Diane not only emerge waving a banner of victory, but she emerged as an encouraging, inspiring, and powerful survivor—a champion.

I Witnessed with excitement as the Lord used her and her circumstances time and time again to reach out with compassion and touch the lives of others, giving them hope and encouragement. With boldness she has stepped out of her comfort zone to allow God to use her life, knowing that everything is part of His perfect will.

I Observe today, Diane diligently standing guard in protecting and strengthening her body. Her battles have produced a trained, equipped, and experienced warrior who knows that health, exercise, love of family and friends, and a strong relationship with her Lord are her weapons of mass destruction against the enemy of cancer.

I Admire my friend who so graciously encouraged me, prayed with me, cried with me, laughed with me, and gave me sound advice in forming my personal plan of attack against my own cancer battle. She is an "inspiring" survivor, a champion, a mentor, and a woman of God's grace.

I Believe Diane has been prepared and inspired through the crucible of cancer to write this timely book. With a heart of compassion, she shares her personal story of battles and victories, desiring to encourage and give hope to those who are currently in their own struggles and for those who will join the fight. I believe this book will accomplish her goal.

CONTENTS

Chapter One

THIS BOOK

I know that not everyone who chooses to read this book has just been diagnosed with cancer. Why you are holding it in your hands or why anyone else might have it in their hands is not by chance. If I had to come up with a reason why we are speaking to one another, I could guess and say that it caught your eye, or that maybe you are looking for advice or comfort. Whatever your reason, life is full of events we want to call "chance," when they really aren't chance at all. All of us go searching for answers when we get our diagnosis of something. In my case it was cancer. In your case it may or may not be called cancer, but whatever your reasons … come on in and I hope I can help.

I decided when writing this book that I wanted to give you my happy ending at the start of my story. I did this because I know that we all need to have our hope reinforced. Like I said above, I know that whatever the reason you opened this cover you need to hear that there is a happy ending. Your heart may feel as if it has stopped because of some devastating news, or in my case, diagnosis. Maybe you can barely catch your breath over the thought of what your future now holds. Maybe you have just received news you thought was reserved for people you don't know. Maybe, it's not about you but someone you know or even love. ... *Stop!* Don't get too far ahead of yourself. If you feel like solid ground has disappeared from under your feet, hang on. There is hope. There is no guarantee for any of us, but there is always hope. Hope from our family and friends. Hope for our plans lived out. Hope for our dreams fulfilled. Hope from our faith that carries us when we can't carry ourselves any further. *Hope.*

So, here's my story with my happy ending first ... my hope.

Chapter Two

A WEDDING

"*H*Mom, I'm engaged!"

"Oh, Ashley, that's wonderful," I said, "Tell me everything."

She began her story, and the words flowed at an amazing rate. Like a rushing stream, she talked, and the flow picked up more and more details. Where? When? How? His proposal. She was happy, unbelievably happy.

My head was swimming with her words. A torrent of thoughts and excitement filled my entire being as I was swept into the current of her words. The river revealed that we had four months to plan a full-scale 300-plus wedding.

Now, I like a party as much as the next person, but this was going to be a monumental feat. My oldest daughter was getting married. Oh my goodness, she was really getting married, and she wanted it to come together in less than four months. Plus … she and the groom had a budget! I knew budgets rarely played well in the planning of weddings.

Practicality started to push me under the surface of her river of words. Worries began swirling around me trying to invade my head and heart. Ashley continued with her story unaware of my concern. *What's the hurry?* I thought as her words continued fast and furious.

Ashley explained her plan and their financial strategy as I struggled to stay floating on the surface. I took a deep breath, smiled, and told myself to listen. *Get a grip, Diane. Remember ... focus on what is good and noble.* Why shouldn't they rush? They had life plans that were looming and they wanted to do them as a married couple. They were looking to make a covenant before God and their families. They were in love. They had been dating for the last four years. *It will be fine,* I told myself. No, it would be fabulous. *I knew how to do this.* I knew how to power through and make the presentation great.

Suddenly, Ashley's words ended just as quickly as they had started, and she told me she would keep me posted. Oh, and she would e-mail me her to-do list. Just as quickly, the call was over, and I was left flopping on the shore like a fish out of water. As quickly as the flood of words had come, they had ended, and from that moment on, time vanished and wedding planning occupied every moment.

Chapter Three

THE HAPPY ENDING

Four months later, I stood there looking out at a sunny day in August 2009. My heart was so full I thought it might burst. Friends and family approached and gave their congratulations. Tables were covered in billowing white and ivory cloths. Chairs were skirted and bowed. The smell of flowers and champagne floated through the air. The clearest blue sky hung above, and the calmest blue lake sat beside. The lawn was manicured to perfection and candles illuminated the silky tents and cast magical shadows across the happy faces.

There on the raised-brick patio, flanked by glowing lanterns, stood my oldest daughter and her new husband. They were laughing and thanking everyone around them. They looked as if they had actually just stepped off the top of their wedding cake. Ashley's piles of soft strawberry curls lay gracefully on her bare shoulders as her new husband in his black tux carefully maneuvered around her dress. At the clink of fine stemware, their eyes met and their lips touched. My husband, Tom, and I and the rest of our children looked on and smiled and laughed.

Again, my breath shortened and I found myself searching my mind, trying to figure out the thoughts that raced through my head. With each thought came a new person hugging and laughing. I was so grateful for each one of them. I thanked them as my eyes continued to focus on the happy couple. The band began to play, and the crowd slowly wandered to the brick-paved dance floor. Soon the couple, my couple, was dancing into dusk.

Slowly, between conversations and dance moves I figured it out. Every fiber of my being was bathed in thankfulness. I was thankful to be alive. I was thankful to my family and friends whose generosity had flowed into this day. I was thankful for all the love that surrounded this moment. But more than anything, I was thankful in my heart to God for His presence in my life and over this blessed event. I was thankful for the journey He had carried me through to get me to this point. This wedding was a life event that I had dreamed of, grieved over, and in my darkest hours of cancer, feared I'd never see for any of my children. This day had proved to be a glorious day and a true testimony to God's grace and His love.

Not too long ago, I had wondered whether I'd be here for life's milestones. You're likely wondering about the future too. I know you probably aren't feeling particularly thankful right now, but you will again. I promise. For me, my daughter's wedding was a blessing when every hope and dream lined up to confirm that there is a plan. This plan isn't one that we are often able to see, or often understand. I will relive this glorious day over and over again in my mind. Cancer had made this moment clearer than I ever could have done on my own.

So, I've been where you are right now. It's a scary, unknown place. Thankfulness is a distant thought right now, but don't think you won't get your own suit of thankfulness no matter what your role is in this current drama playing out. I will tell you that it is a process. A journey you are now forced to take. A journey into who you really are, what you really believe, and what you really want out of this time you've been given, called life. It's time to take a look at the impact of hearing you or your loved one has been diagnosed with cancer.

This is my story.

Chapter Four

THE LUMP

*L*et's go back now to May 1999. It started in the shower. I was standing there planning my day and doing shower things when I felt it. At least, I thought I felt something. My body stiffened. Did I? … I felt around again. Yep, it felt like something was there. It felt squishy but then again slightly firm. Was that really that unusual? Had it been there all along and this was the first time I had come across it? I racked my brain trying to figure out what this spot could be from. Had I bumped myself? Was I hormonal? Was I imagining it?

I finished my shower and tried to put this discovery out of my mind. However, every day when I entered the shower, I played around with this spot. For two weeks I verified its existence. Every shower was a new attempt to identify and explain what the reality of the situation was. Was it a lump or wasn't it? I told myself repeatedly that I was being ridiculous. There probably wasn't even anything really there. I would wish it away each day and move through my routine, ignoring my discovery!

I knew that a few weeks later I had a routine office visit scheduled with my doctor. It had been placed on my calendar long before this discovery. It was time for my annual. If you are a woman reading this book, you know that an "annual" is code for that extremely awkward visit with your doctor. This visit is where you leave all modesty at the door and try to make polite conversation about your physical concerns or issues. This visit is generally the visit that most women dread. Now, I know some women don't mind at all, but I would say it's about 80/20 in the "dread" department.

I decided I would mention this spot to my doctor during my checkup. Of course, I knew it would probably be nothing. There was no logical reason to think this small thing was anything to worry about. I refused to even entertain the idea of anything serious. The thought that I would have breast cancer was preposterous. Did I just think "breast cancer"? *Don't be silly,* I told myself. I decided to eliminate the thought from my mind and move on with my day. I knew I didn't have time to stew over this. If I didn't get moving, my day would move on without me.

My day, like most of my days, is organized chaos. I didn't need an overly dramatic idea to come along and disrupt it. I already had the appointment scheduled, and I would mention to the doctor what "I thought" I "might" have felt in the shower. It was settled.

Chapter Five

DOCTOR'S APPOINTMENT

*I*t was now approximately two weeks since my discovery in the shower, and time for the doctor's appointment. I entered the office and went through the usual sign-in procedures and paperwork. Yes—same address, telephone, and emergency contact information. I sat patiently until they called my name.

All ladies know the next phase of these appointments: "Step on the scale please." "Oh, okay," I replied, as hopeful thoughts rushed through my head. Whew, not bad.

"Have a seat and we'll get your blood pressure. ... Looks good," the nurse said with a cheery smile. Question, question, question ... "Oh really? Make sure you mention that to the doctor."

"Absolutely, first thing," I said.

"Okay. There's the gown; he'll be in shortly."

"Thanks," I said.

So I hopped up on the table and waited for the doctor. This is always when time seems to stand still. You look around the room and notice every detail, like how the wallpaper is lifting at a seam or that the magazines in the rack are at least one holiday too late. My eyes were drawn to the breast self-exam poster. I wondered if women actually did that on a consistent basis. Is anyone that predictable and organized? I wasn't. Oh sure, I wanted to be, but usually I was trying to cram ten minutes of work into two minutes of time. Then, my thoughts stopped as the door opened.

"Hello, Diane."

"Hello, how are you?" I said

"Good, how are you doing?" he said.

"Good. Oh, I'm supposed to mention this spot I found."

"Oh, okay we'll take a look," he said as he laid down my chart.

He washed his hands and started the normal process. I'm not going into any more detail here. If you are a woman, you know the drill.

We moved through polite conversation about my health, and I shared more detail of my discovery in the shower. He didn't seem alarmed and informed me that it was good I was having him check it out. He then proceeded to examine the designated breast.

"Yes, I feel it. Doesn't seem to be bigger than a dime," the doctor said. Then he reassured me, "Eighty percent of all breast lumps are benign. However," he added, "you are thirty-nine, and I don't see here that you've ever had a mammogram. I think it would be a good idea for you to have one, and let's see what it shows."

"Sure," I said.

He scheduled a mammogram for the very next day. I really hate to elaborate on what a mammogram is, but I will. Imagine scooping every spare bit of flesh on your body onto a tray, only to have it squished as thin as possible. I mean crepe thin. This is necessary to get a clear picture of all the tissue. I will just say that

I do believe mammograms should be followed by a ceremony recognizing your heroic efforts and amazing endurance, and should possibly be followed by a ribbon-pinning ceremony.

After all of this effort, the results were inconclusive, so my doctor moved on to ordering an ultrasound. "Nothing to be alarmed at, but we want to be sure," he said.

"Of course," I said.

Well, the ultrasound revealed the lump. It couldn't hide any longer. The tech assured me that this looked nothing like what breast cancer should look like. Oh, I thought, more confirmation that this was probably nothing. The tech repeated that most breast lumps are benign and that we just had to go through the basics. There probably was nothing to worry about. Everybody kept telling me there probably was nothing to worry about. However, the more they said that there was probably nothing to worry about, the more I started to think about what not to worry about.

At the end of the week, the doctor still had no conclusive results, but there definitely was a lump, and since it didn't belong there, we needed to remove it. I knew this meant surgery. It still didn't make too much of an impact on me. I wasn't going to put the cart before the horse. I was only thirty-nine. I would choose to hang on to the positive comments of the doctor. He scheduled the surgical biopsy with a local surgeon. I just wanted to get this over with so I could get it off my calendar and whatever it was out of my breast. It couldn't come quick enough for me.

Chapter Six

BIOPSY

$\mathcal{M}$y appointment time had come. Tom and I went to the hospital, and I was readied for the biopsy. I was nervous, but I was telling myself to stay positive. There really wasn't any reason not to be optimistic. Everyone had repeatedly reassured me that this was typical procedure, nothing out of the ordinary. Tom was sitting by my bedside trying to keep my mind busy with other matters. It didn't work. We had been married long enough that I could tell he was nervous too.

As I was sitting and waiting a question popped into my head: Do you trust? Did I trust? Did we trust? *Yes,* I answered in my mind. I knew I trusted my God, my faith. I also knew that trust doesn't mean "not scared." Was Jesus scared? He had to be. The Bible tells us that He had sweat drops of blood before going to the cross. I comforted myself with the thought that no matter what the outcome, He would be there with us. I trusted that.

Soon the nurses came for me. Tom and I prayed quietly with each other and then we each said "love you and see you later." We smiled with love in our eyes and hope in our hearts. I can't say I remember much after that. I do remember waking to pain.

Not much pain, but a feeling that something had happened while I was asleep under the anesthesia.

As I was lying in the recovery bed, ironically or obviously, I had no idea what was happening outside my door. Tom was still waiting out in the hall for me to come out of recovery, when Laura and her husband passed by. These were close friends of ours going through breast cancer. They had spotted Tom and were asking him about my procedure and how he and I were doing.

I had no idea that the possible results of breast cancer were visiting with my husband in the hallway. Tom was getting a good look at his and my possible future. Cancer had wreaked its havoc on this dear couple and Tom was standing there with cancer looking him in the face through the eyes of our friends.

Seeing Laura had sent Tom's mind racing: racing to his life with a wife who has cancer; then to life with no wife; then to a life with four children to parent alone. His mind was filled with the thoughts of a life so different and a change too heartbreaking to comprehend. I was unaware that my husband had seen his possible future in the hall. I should've known something had happened by the look on his face when he came into the room. I didn't.

Chapter Seven

LAURA

*L*aura had been diagnosed years earlier with breast cancer, and it seemed to us, her friends, that she was losing her battle. She had been spending the last year bravely dealing with her mortality. She had been very open about her situation and we all admired her resolve. Tom and I had often spoken about Laura's and her husband's strength and poise.

Laura was a "breast friend" before I even knew I needed one. It wouldn't be long after my diagnosis that Laura would lose her battle with cancer. Laura had shared with me that she had found her peace and her voice in her cancer. Cancer does give you a voice. Sometimes the voice is a whisper or sometimes it is a scream. Laura had talked about her need to share with others this experience called cancer. Laura's final use of her voice was to give a prerecorded speech at her own funeral. At her service, her church family sat staring at the lifeless shell, while we listened to her life-giving speech. She told us about her walk with the Lord, her battle with cancer, and her love for all those who had surrounded her. She had no regrets and only love in her heart. It was as if she were right there with us, smiling at us, gently showing us ourselves and how much she had appreciated our love.

Throughout her battle and regardless of her condition, Laura had always led me and others down the road of optimism with her kind words. Laura even used her funeral to lift the rest of us. You get to decide what you use your "voice" for. Laura used hers to speak encouragement into my life and many others. I am eternally grateful for the investment she made in me. I appreciated and loved her.

Laura had made peace with her diagnosis and her God. I know He comes to each of us in a personal way. If you haven't found Him yet, this could be your wake-up call to look.

Chapter Eight

YOU HAVE CANCER

*T*he doctor came into my room with Tom. The doctor did all of the talking … I should have known it wasn't good. Tom's face had a look I had never seen before. He looked like someone had let the air out of him. That look worried me instantly. I searched his face and then the doctor's. *Just say it. No … don't say it. I don't want to hear it. Tom, do not let them say it.*

There was no stopping what was to come next.

"Diane, I'm sorry to have to tell you that we took the lump and, we are absolutely sure that it is cancer." *What? Wait a minute. I have cancer? I'm married … I have four kids who, by the way, were nursed for a year each. Wasn't that preventative medicine number one? I'm only thirty-nine years old. No one in my family has had breast cancer. I have five sisters and one brother, all cancer free. I have a wonderful healthy mother. I'm in the middle of all these healthy siblings. This can't be right. I'm not even at risk. This is ridiculous. The test must be wrong. That can happen. I've heard of it happening.* I could feel my heart racing. My mind was going in a hundred different directions.

I could feel my life changing in that instant. Cancer had made a mistake. God was making a mistake. I don't have time for this.

I don't want to make time for this. Why? Why now? Why me? Why was this happening? What had I done wrong? *Cancer happens to other people,* I thought. *Why?* Tom and the doctor faded from my view as tears filled my eyes. This can't be. I could feel my anger rising as hot tears stained my face and gown. Tom put his face to mine, and we wept together. I laid there with no place to run to. All of my life's coping skills landed wet on my husband and my hospital bed.

Chapter Nine

GOD

I know I am a person of faith. I treasure my relationship with Jesus, but all the life-giving Scripture I held so close in my heart suddenly seemed distant. I desperately wanted to have a sense of purpose and security in this situation that was happening to me. Honestly, I have to say I wasn't immediately able to draw on God's strength. I thought I would be able to pull that power out of my pocket and hang it around my neck like a badge. When I needed it most, I was having trouble resting in my faith. Scriptures flashed through my head, but none seemed to take hold or comfort me. Nothing could comfort me.

It was only when the thought that this could happen to anyone struck me like a lightning bolt that I began to focus. This was happening *for* me not *to* me. I knew that God was no respecter of persons. *There has to be a plan in all of this,* I thought. My agony still raged repeatedly after this personal revelation, and repeatedly I had to remind myself that God knows the plans He has for us. But, at least I could rest in the fact that God chooses to use each of us for His purpose not ours. I had to remember who was running this show.

Chapter Ten

TELLING EVERYONE

om and I told our kids that weekend. We sat them down as a group. My oldest, Ashley, was twelve. Tommy was ten. Hillary was six and Dane was five. I don't really know what I expected, but what I got was pretty calm. Ashley seemed determined to take this in stride and keep things moving along. Tommy was reassuring. Hillary and Dane were six and five, which pretty much explains their reaction. I might as well have been telling them we were having chicken for dinner. Dinner would have been far more relevant information to them, but they took their cue from the older children and listened. Tom kept their focus by insisting how serious this would be for our family. I knew my two oldest were being very brave and my two youngest were too young to understand the weight of what had been said.

It was a lot harder to tell our parents and siblings. Parents were worried, and siblings reached out with concern. It caught everyone off guard—I think especially my five sisters. I knew they would be now looking at their "femininity" very differently. My brother was reassuring. They all expressed their love and caring.

That felt good because, honestly, it isn't something we take time to show each other often enough. There was an outpouring of love from my parents and Tom's parents.

Sadly, they all knew what I knew. Now, there would be a family history of cancer. I had changed all of their lives the instant I was diagnosed. I was making them a statistic without their permission. I felt sad for that, for them, for my daughters.

You may not even know that yet, but if you've been diagnosed with cancer, you have changed not only your life but the lives of everyone related to you. Some people may not be very appreciative of that fact. No matter what anyone thinks about how you've impacted them, you have to move on through your journey and put their worries aside.

Tom and I also told our church family and close friends. For them, it was a rallying cry to get to work. Various ministries were called and arrangements were made. These people were accustomed to being pulled into service. They knew what they could do: prayer, support, and food.

I also told my coworkers. This news was going to change how I did my job. I especially remember telling Char. She embraced me and cried with me and told me she loved me like I was one of her own. Char had lost her dearest friend to breast cancer already. I knew it was especially hard on her to relive the horrible loss breast cancer had inflicted on her. I knew Char would be a soft place for me to land during this time, and I still treasure her friendship to this day.

I strongly recommend a church family and calling on those friends who will hold your hair back and help you put on your socks. They will be there not for themselves, but for you. These friends share that quiet confidence that no matter what the circumstances, "God is on His throne." These people are the treasures in my life. Their prayers and consoling faith lifted me at every stage. They kept me going forward and still do to this day. Like I said, I strongly recommend a Savior that is our hope, a church family that wraps its arms around you, and friends who love you in spite of yourself.

Chapter Eleven

THE REACTION

Okay, I already told you how my kids reacted—enough said. Friends were different. This took me by surprise. Like bad news, cancer news travels fast. Soon the door to my house would open and some people I hadn't seen or heard from for a long time would suddenly appear. A few well-meaning friends would offer their words of support and then switch into what seemed almost like a pre-funeral service. Unintentionally, I was hearing about the future without me in it. Ironically, the next thing I knew, I was reassuring my visitors that they would be okay. Life had to go on. Thanks for stopping by. ... Blah! Blah! Blah!

After a couple of these visits of emotional meltdown, I decided I had to look at myself from a living perspective. *I'm not dead!* I screamed inside my head. I knew I had to decide who I could surround myself with. I appreciated the caring, but I needed positive, uplifting support. I needed help out of the well not into it. That core of friends revealed itself. I clung to them and relied on them for the strength I needed. Let's just say, their get well cards had legs, and they often knew my needs before I even asked.

They didn't just put me in their prayers. They called and asked to pray with me.

Now don't get me wrong. I appreciated all the love and caring that came my way, but I knew that I needed warriors. I'm a realist, and I had to look at myself like someone who had a future. I purposefully decided that no words of misplaced encouragement coated with despair would be allowed to make a home in my brain. I purposed to stay strong and positive. I would somehow make it through all of this and take the fear of the unknown head-on.

Sure, I was entering what felt like a dark tunnel, and I couldn't see the end. There was no prelaid track for my train, but it was going to be a moving train, not one of those abandoned ones in the yard. I knew that I had others in their prayer closets praying for me, and that would give me the freedom to fight. All those prayers would be neatly packed into my suitcase so that I could use them on my journey.

It was the first time in my life I found myself hesitant to enter my own prayer closet, but I could literally feel the prayers of those who loved me. It was the most amazing feeling I had ever experienced in the prayer department. These prayer warriors were allowed to board my train anytime they wanted. I knew cancer was going to be a daily battle, and I chose to be the conductor of how this train would leave the station. I didn't have the medical strategy yet, but I had the most important part of the fight nailed down!

Chapter Twelve

LIFE & SCHEDULING CANCER

$\mathcal{R}$ight about now, I'd like to tell you that the world stopped. Of course, everyone and everything focused on me. I'd like to tell you that people surrounded me 24-7. I had endless love and care and didn't have to lift a finger. I could tell you I was the complete focus of everyone's attention, and their goal was to get me well again. I could tell you that my husband dropped everything he was doing, even his business and family concerns. I could tell you that my kids vowed to pick up everything they owned and put it where it actually belonged. Meals were provided. My house never got dirty. All family disputes were solved and never mentioned again. Yeah right! I could tell you that, but that didn't happen. Not even close. Cancer or no cancer, life goes on. Cancer doesn't stop the parade of your life. Cancer just hops on one of the floats and starts waving. One of the things I discovered is that cancer is waving at *you* and not the crowd. So, even though the parade continues, cancer makes you pay attention to it.

My life included a husband and four children. Every day was a new race to run. If you are like me, your race of chaos has a beginning, middle, and rarely an end. Even so, I had this chaos organized. Handling chaos had been something I perfected even before a husband and children were added to my life. At least, that's what I thought. Most of us fool ourselves with that idea. Somehow, I had convinced myself that things were subject to my plans. But, cancer comes along and forces you to sit down, be still, and listen. Not head-nodding, grocery-list-making, microwave-punching, job-organizing listening. Instead, eyes-focused, no-other-sound-but-your-heart-beating listening. The kind of listening we try to keep under control. Why? Because it can take you down so many roads you don't want to go. Roads that we'd never go down unless someone or something grabbed hold of us and kicked us along that way. Cancer was forcing me down that road, and it was forcing me to make changes to my life.

My first priority had always been to take care of my family, and cancer was changing how I was going to do that. Doesn't matter what I had planned. Doesn't matter who's in your life or who's not. Doesn't matter how you thought things were supposed to go. Cancer forces us and our families down that new road and off our own chaotic highway—often into the care of strangers. Some of these strangers will know a lot about us, our family, and even our body. Some of these strangers will have "Dr." in front of their name and some will be trying to navigate the same cancer highway. More importantly, cancer will shove you into the "rest" of your God. A God we so carefully claim, until our lives depend on it.

Chapter Thirteen

MY HUSBAND

$\mathcal{A}$t the time of this life-altering news, my husband had assumed full control of his father's business. My husband was a third generation logger. His dad and his grandfather had established a very successful logging business. I had married a very dedicated and hard working logger who loved what he did for a living. If you live anywhere where there are a lot of trees, you probably know what a logger does. If not, I'll clarify and you use your imagination. Definition of a logger: gone. And I mean gone a lot.

There is always a new tree to cut, move, and get paid for. This frantic schedule puts food on your table, clothes on your back, and a roof over your head. Of course, there is always a truck that needs fixing, and that usually happens at 2 a.m. or when the church play is scheduled. Never does the truck break down when you've just finished praying and getting your thought life on track. I've come to believe that we all have some type of logger or broken semi in our life. Maybe it's you that's the logger or maybe you're just broken. We learn to function no matter what the conditions or the circumstances. So, good or bad, this was my family's life and I embraced it. I told myself I was fine with it. I had a lot of control because of this lifestyle. I decided what happened in my household. My husband had a job to do and so did I. We both had a schedule to keep.

My husband's takeover of the family logging business was a dramatic personal and financial event, and it was still unclear how it was going to shake out for my family. Tom hadn't refined the process of running a family business on his own yet.

My father-in-law had been diagnosed with a condition that would eventually rob him of his role as fully functioning logger and overall superman. He was told, "You can't drive, and soon you won't be able to do anything for yourself." My husband had been living with this devastating news. His whole family was trying to cope with this development. I was worried about Tom, who was already running from point A to point B as fast as he could, and now cancer had been thrown onto his pile. I felt so responsible for the additional burden, but there was nothing I could do about it. I wanted to do something about it. I didn't want him to have to handle another issue but I knew he would have to handle it. I had my own points A and B to get to. I'd have to handle cancer.

My husband and I never sat down and came up with a plan for handling my cancer. I could tell by his demeanor that he never doubted that I would handle it, but I knew he was afraid my strength wouldn't be enough. I could see the concern and sadness that would blanket his face. I hated being the reason for this new hardship. I'd always hated letting others down. I knew he was already overwhelmed with the challenges that kept showing up on his doorstep. His plate was completely full.

It always seemed to me that most men, like my husband, figure that their role is to "fix" a problem. I know Tom wanted to fix my cancer. I know he wanted to make me better with all his heart. He desperately wanted to fix it. He couldn't fix this. He couldn't control this situation and neither could I.

I needed to talk and to hear all my fears bouncing off the walls. I needed to see them as ridiculous once they were voiced and to run down every avenue of pain and doubt. I wanted to not have to make sense, to not worry about reactions, or care about how I was impacting others. Talking was what I needed because nobody, not even a loving husband could fix this. I discovered you have to process through cancer. I knew I had girlfriends who would listen. You can't fix cancer. You can follow directions and pray. I knew my husband would always be willing to listen, but the pain cancer was inflicting on him was enough. I chose to unload on my friends and God.

I tried to spread my need accordingly. That way, I wouldn't impose too heavily on any one person. Do you go through your day like that? Constantly, I was trying to minimize my impact on others. Constantly anticipating what kind of reaction I'd get? Tucking my pain and fears away when the situation was too uncomfortable for others? I knew I was being forced into new territory. I'd have to lean when I wasn't used to leaning and continue to surrender to God's plan. My husband would have to do the same. I'd try to spare Tom as much as I could. I knew what he was dealing with, and I didn't want to burden him more.

Here's where I suggest you refine the process. Share, talk, … look into the eyes of your loved ones and bring them along with you. You can't protect them, so let them in, because the plan isn't just for you. I didn't know that then. You probably think this is all about you. It is your body for heaven's sake. But, your body is such a small part of what is happening to you. Everything is going to change. You're going to change. Not little changes like your eye shadow color, or briefs or bikini, but soul-wrenching, fall-to-the-ground, wanting-to-stop-the-pain change. Guess what? Your loved ones will change too. They just won't have the physical scars to prove it. But the scars will be there, and scars are okay. They mark where you've been and influence where you are choosing to go. They will reflect the control you've lost and the freedom you've found.

Because really, isn't control a funny idea? It is to me now. Now I know control is an illusion most of us operate under until something like cancer comes along and smacks our control in the face. God knows we were never in control. He tells us to trust Him. He tells us He knows the plan He has for us. He watches and waits for us to give in to the plan, knowing all along that we don't have a choice. He knows that some will get with the program immediately; others, not so quickly. But, He waits for each one of us.

Chapter Fourteen

KIDS

My kids, like most kids, were busy. So, busy times four, means really busy! The kids were dutifully enrolled in church and activities that would produce loving, upright, socially responsible citizens. I had them on track. They didn't always cooperate with my track, but it was a track going somewhere and I felt good about that. Besides, kids aren't supposed to keep the track clutter free.

Each of my children was laying down their tracks for life, and I was very proud of them. If, you're a mother (or a pet owner, or a gardener, or whatever is meaningful in your life), you cherish your children. You love the way they are moving along from one station of life to another. You cheer with them, cry with them, and of course, think other people are doing a better job with their children and their track (at least that's what I always thought). Guess what? It's not true and it doesn't matter anyway. My track had great love and presentation and I wasn't going to beat myself up over comparing tracks. I knew this was going to have to change some. Cancer was going to force me to send some things in for repairs and storage.

Now, you might have kids … you might not. You might have a husband or someone interesting in your life, and you might not. But, I know your life is full of your stuff and your people, and you are busy. Well, like I said, cancer says that some of this stuff is going to have to wait. Unlike, your husband and his concerns, your kids and their needs, your father-in-law and his illness, or your boss, you don't get to zone out on cancer. Cancer forces you to look it in the eye and take time for it. My kids picked up on this quickly. It didn't stop them from being kids, but it did stop me from being the conductor at times. I didn't like that. I still don't. So I learned the art of prioritizing. I learned that really listening was far more important than running. I realized that anyone could do the daily running, but only I could be the mother listening. Turns out, it's always about the people in our lives, not the stuff we do, and usually my kids just wanted me to be able to pay attention.

Chapter Fifteen

BATTLE PLAN

*O*kay, so here comes my big decision. Maybe you have the same decisions to make. You are about to go to war. How are you going to wage the battle? Crawling into a cave and ignoring it is not an option. Besides, if you have kids or anyone else who cares for you, they'll find you, cancer or no cancer.

Step one: I had made an appointment with the doctor the following Monday to answer the treatment questions. Now, like most things in life, this didn't go smoothly. Apparently, my records had not reached or even been requested for the next destination.

Step two: I thought to myself what does this mean? Because, after you recover from your numb stage your senses are in high alert! You are facing life and death, and there is no room for mistakes.

Step three: I started asking questions because I'm a questioning girl. You can verify that with my husband if you'd like. I know there have been plenty of times when he would have liked to just reach over and gently cover my mouth. Regardless, I went into detective mode. I asked the doctor point blank, "If I were your wife, would you be satisfied with this course or would you seek additional advice?" He paused. I could see the wheels of diplomacy turning. He complimented the proficiency of the local facility and stated that local care was available. I listened, and I knew in my heart I needed to be where there were women like me. Thirty-nine-year-old women who wanted doctors who were pushing the envelope and on the cutting edge of technology (no pun intended).

Step four: I took action. I chose Mayo Clinic. Be on the alert for the red flags. They'll pop up every now and again. It's up to you to pay attention. I took the fact that my records had not reached their destination as verification for my decision. I figured it was God's way of nudging me on to something else. I trusted Him and His nudges.

Chapter Sixteen

MAYO

*I*t was at Mayo that I learned how I would spend a good portion of my upcoming schedule. The doctors laid out very specifically what they would do for me and what they expected from me. The words fell out of their mouths quickly and easily. These were the generals I would be taking orders from.

The pathology report showed grade 4, nuclear grade 2, invasive, adenocarcinoma with mixed ductal and lobular features. Lobular carcinoma had a slightly higher incidence of occurrence in the contralateral breast ... which didn't preclude breast conservation. The words flowed into my brain like sand, and I could feel my head filling up. Soon, I was like an hourglass, ready to be turned over and started again. I felt like I needed to ask my husband to flip me so I could go on listening. I found I couldn't take mental notes like I would of in any other situation. Thank goodness my husband could help decipher this new language. I was weirdly detached from the meaning of all this even though this was my body that was being discussed. I did pick up that my physical appearance could be forever altered and that my self-esteem was on the proverbial butcher block with the options that were being discussed. I thanked God that I had Tom's extra ears and heart to classify the information in a thorough manner since I couldn't seem to clear the sand out. Even with his help and discernment, I can see now some of my wrong thinking. Because no matter how much information you're given you have never been through cancer before, and it still comes down to you saying yes or no to all the options placed before you. Naturally, your decisions are full of all your preconceived ideas about who you are or think you are.

Take your time and learn. Ask and ask again.

Chapter Seventeen

TREATMENT

*M*y first treatment was to have more surgery. My doctor gave me the choice of a wide local excision and auxiliary lymph node dissection or a full mastectomy. In layman's terms: a lumpectomy or removal of the whole breast. Sounds fun huh? The doctor said I was a good candidate for either procedure. Well, that was comforting. What if you're not a good candidate for either? Where do you go from there? Honestly, I don't know and I'm glad I didn't have to know. Fortunately, I was a "good candidate."

Following the layout of the options, I spoke with the oncologist about chemotherapy. Of course, I had lots of questions. One of my biggest concerns was the rest of my female parts. Could they be infected? The doctor told me that everything would be thoroughly investigated, and he arranged for me to have all the necessary tests to check out this possibility.

I'd never heard any of this stuff before. I'm sure most people haven't. My advice is don't be intimidated. Find out what you need to so you can put your mind at rest. If it's one hundred questions, ask. You need to do what you have to do to be at peace with the process.

After everything, I decided to keep my breast, remove the lump and some lymph nodes, and go through chemotherapy and radiation. I could live with that decision, and my husband was very supportive of what I wanted to do. I sensed his relief now that the decision was made. His goal was always to get me back to health as soon as possible, and there was no question that he would be with me every step of the way.

When I got home, I sought the counsel of a person I didn't know very well but who had been referred to me as a breast cancer survivor. Her name is Sandi. She took my call and listened patiently as I unfolded my story and bombarded her with questions. I'm sure I made an overwhelming first impression. She described her own experience and took me through the process. That one conversation elevated my confidence and calmed my fears. I had an idea of what to expect, and I knew that conversation opened the door to a full-blown confidante and friend. Sandi was there to answer all my questions and is to this day.

Chapter Eighteen

SURGERY

Within a week, I was back at Mayo, and waiting to be rolled into surgery. There wasn't anything particularly special about prep for surgery. The usual IV, allergy questions, warm blankets, and worried looks exchanged between loved ones. My loved one was trying to be especially upbeat and casual. I wasn't trying to be anything but focused on getting it over as quickly as possible.

Once in surgery, the doctor removed the lump and some lymph nodes. I awoke knowing that a great deal had happened while I was asleep. I was sore and groggy, and across my body was a layer of tubes that I didn't have before. It was like being an alien in my own body. I was afraid to move. Actually, I don't think I could've moved even if I wanted to. One thought kept running through my head: *I had completed one step of the journey.* Doctors showed up to explain what had been done and what to expect. They said that the surgery had basically disfigured a third of my right breast, but the good news of the day was that the cancer had not spread to any lymph nodes. However, they were all removed from under my right arm as a precaution. For the first time, I actually had the feeling that this may not kill me, and I really did feel like this was good news regardless of the whole disfigurement thing.

Tom reassured me that everything went as planned. I could tell he was relieved to have me one step closer to better, and so was I. I would only be given two weeks before I would start chemotherapy. Tom and I were told that I could get my chemo treatment done closer to home. This would save us from having to drive all the way to Mayo and back. That was a relief, since Mayo was a good six to seven hours from my home. It wasn't at all practical or possible to drive back and forth for chemo. The doctors reassured us that chemo was something that could be managed from anywhere that had the appropriate facilities.

Chapter Nineteen

CHEMO

$\mathcal{T}$he plan was that I would undergo four rounds of chemotherapy. I was told all of the side effects that would accompany my treatment. They said that one of the most noticeable would be that my hair would fall out. Okay, not the best news, but compared to cancer, definitely not the worst news. I told myself I could do this.

Tom and I drove down to my first chemo appointment in Green Bay, Wisconsin. This was about a two-hour drive from our home. Everything is "about one to two hours away in the U.P. of Michigan." (Inside joke for all the Yoopers reading this book.) I was glad to have Tom with me. We tried to keep things positive and focused. I kept telling myself that this was just another step in my healing. I knew all of this was taking me down the road to restored health. Nothing else would be acceptable to me.

When we arrived at the office, we stepped through the door of a whole new world. This office was filled with people who looked sick—I mean, really sick. I knew I didn't look 100 percent, but I still felt strong. It was an odd revelation that I now belonged in this environment. I would be coming to this place where people were fighting for their lives. I would be fighting for my life too. I told myself I didn't want to get too comfortable with this. I had a job to do: get better.

"Diane Casperson," the nurse said.

"That's me."

The nurses were ready for me. They were very nice. Not overly concerned, not completely indifferent. Mostly, they all had knowing looks on their faces. I was, after all, just another cancer patient.

I was placed in what would be my chemo chair and given an IV. The nurse quickly explained the process and moved on with the task at hand. First of all, let me tell you that prior to the chemo going in, they give you steroids. These are meant to prepare your body for the drain that chemo was going to put it through. So, in go the steroids before the poison. It's odd to think that you are purposely allowing a stranger to pour poison into your veins of your own free will. My whole life was previously spent avoiding toxic chemicals. Now, I was purposely allowing a stranger to fill me up with the stuff. Well … one toxic step towards defeating my enemy, I told myself. I knew that they would be giving me enough chemo to "just about kill me." What if it did kill me? No … that would definitely discourage future visits. I reassured myself that they knew when to stop.

Quickly it was all over and they sent Tom and me on our way. "Bye," the nurses said.

"Bye," I repeated back like we were going to have coffee next time. *Okay, hope I don't die before I see you next,* I thought. Say hi to the family … nope, there was none of that.

Soon someone else was taking my place in the chemo chair. *Nice.* It was a very disconcerting situation to be in, but I knew I was just a part of their job. These medical people did this every day. This was how it had to be. I decided to look at chemo as just another part of my job right now. I told myself I wouldn't let the absolute horror and emotion of it all take over my mind. I even threw in a "See ya next time," for good measure. They all smiled. Those in the waiting room didn't have the same sunny response. I'm not sure they even heard me. I asked myself if I had heard anything while I was sitting there. The only thing I could remember was my name being called. Yep … just my name.

Tom and I were on our way home. We were both relieved to have the first visit over. I convinced myself and Tom that this was manageable. How awful could it be? I didn't really feel any differently than I had before. I told Tom, "I bet they make it sound worse than it is, to prepare you for your downtime." He shook his head and concentrated on the road. As he was driving, I was starting to feel energized.

Well, in case you've never been on a steroid, let me tell you, it was an experience. I wasn't expecting to feel like doing anything after being shot up with poison, but that's where the steroids come in. I don't think I'd ever had that much energy in my entire life. This is obviously all designed to get you caught up on your housework and any other projects you had been putting off. I was like a bee readying the hive. I felt like this was the cleanest my house had ever been. Did I mention that I had enormous amounts of energy? I buzzed and buzzed and cleaned and cleaned. My nest had never been so organized. I had a new understanding of why people would use these meds for other purposes. Honestly, this is something I would never have had empathy for in the past. Cancer had exposed me to the cleaning frenzy of steroids. However, don't take this as an endorsement, because the pain of cancer isn't worth a clean house. Besides, it's necessary, because once chemo starts, you don't care if your dust bunnies have turned into cattle and taken over the ranch. I'm sure doctors must have discussed this in the lounge and decided steroids were a must to start the process.

Then, right on schedule, I could feel the poison start to work. Within a couple of days, I had the cancer flu. Take H1N1 and put cancer in front of it. I told myself this wasn't so bad. Excuse me while I throw up. I knew this was it … this was when push came to shove, and I decided to shove back.

I kept working my couple of days a week. I decided I'd had worse cases of the flu than this. Of course, I would have to rest when necessary, but I wouldn't lay down for this fight. I knew I had a mighty God!

Many people commented to me how good I looked and how well I appeared to be handling all of this. Well, I didn't really have any idea of how I was supposed to look or handle cancer, but I knew that people were praying for me. I could feel it. I still can't explain that feeling. It was probably the time in my life when I actually prayed the least and yet felt the closest to my God. He was all around me. It wasn't my strength that carried me; it was His. I knew my friends and family were petitioning for me. They told me over and over, and I believed, I trusted, I felt peace. Again, I knew that God was no respecter of persons. His Word told me that He would walk me through this entire thing called cancer.

Chapter Twenty

LOSING MY HAIR

M y hair didn't fall out right away. I knew I could will it not to fall out. I'd be the first cancer patient not to lose my hair. The doctors said it would take about two weeks for my hair to fall out. I was approaching the two-week mark and feeling very confident about my ability to keep my hair rooted. But like always, practicality took over. I decided I had better get a hat just in case. If they actually turned out to be right, I should be prepared. Off I went to Wal-Mart to look at hats. Nobody could tell I wasn't just shopping for hats. There were no signs of cancer showing up, so I started looking through the hat supply. I finally found one that spoke to my personality and thought I'd try it on. Not bad—not bad at all. Actually, I liked it. This hat would do, if needed. I took the hat off and prepared to head to the register. My heart sank. The hat was full of my hair. This took me by surprise. There was no way to put the hat back now even if I didn't like it. My hair had claimed it. I again headed for the register and purchased my first public piece of cancer clothing. I immediately headed home.

As the evening progressed, my hair continued to come out in my hands in clumps. Clumps that made my head look like an unfinished patchwork quilt. I knew there would eventually be no way to style around bare patches. I mean, how do you explain the sun shining off of bare scalp? As usual, I came to the most effective and efficient decision I could. There was nothing to do but take charge. I'd shave my head in the morning. There, I decided. This way, I would be in charge of the process. I liked to find ways to control the uncontrollable. I did that a lot. I also decided to include a dear friend in this process. Practicality required that someone be able to navigate around my scalp skillfully with a razor. I knew every inch of the rest of the razor areas on my body, but not my scalp. I know some men do this all the time. For me, this was new territory. I summoned the woman I felt could handle the job. This was my dear friend, Diane. I didn't know she was going to bring her husband … my pastor. We all know that pastors are called to help in all sorts of situations. I welcomed his compassion as his wife, my friend, helped me to carefully shave off the remaining bit of my womanly crown. They both tried to put a happy face on the situation. I was appreciative of her attempt to lighten the mood and of her shaving skills. I could feel every stroke being done with love. Diane and I cried, hugged, and laughed together, surrounded by the discarded remnants of my hair. This woman had been and is a part of my soul for eternity, and she's at the top of the list of "breast friends."

Don't think that your hair is going to be easy to part with? It isn't. I don't care how short you've worn your hair or how empowered you think you are. Maybe you've never been happy with your hair. Maybe it's too thin, or curly, or frizzy, or grey, or whatever. But guess what? It's there. Unless you are the new girl in the *Star Trek* movie, you're going to miss it. I was surprised how I had clung to the thought that I'd be the first cancer patient not to lose my hair. I mean, a good haircut could conceal a multitude of issues, and I was hoping it might even hide the trauma of cancer. Nope. I lost my hair; I wasn't the exception to the rule. The whole world would see my bald head and the telltale sign that I had cancer. There would be no "slight-of-hair" for me. No denying to strangers that I wasn't 100 percent. No matter how big my smile, I knew the bald head would overpower it.

Chapter Twenty-One

WHAT TO DO ABOUT YOUR BALD HEAD

ooking in the mirror, I saw a cancer patient staring back at me. It was decision time again. Should I go with a wig or a hat? Some people are brave enough to go through life bald. I wasn't sure if I had that kind of strength. First, I didn't want the looks or questions if possible. Second, having no hair would likely make me cold. Hair is definitely a lot warmer than no hair. Third, it could be interesting to have a new hairstyle for a while.

I must tell you that this decision making was occurring without my husband's input. My husband had left for a business trip prior to the loss of my hair. Before he left, I still had my hair exactly where it was supposed to be. He hadn't witnessed the tears and clumps falling in the bathroom and on my bed and all over my clothes, or the shaving of my head. So, I was going to test him with my new look when he returned home. This would give me an accurate assessment of where he was in this whole cancer process. I decided to go without hair for his initial return and then consult him on the options.

When Tom walked through the front door, I was standing at the top of our stairway— in all my bald-head glory! Tom set his stuff down and looked.

"Wow, how are you?" he said.

"Wow? That's all?" I said.

"I'm bald!"

"So? You look great." He didn't care. *He really didn't care.* He had the same loving look on his face as always. What I did see was his relief. He was relieved to see me standing at the top of the stairs; relieved that I wasn't slumped somewhere falling to pieces, wallowing in self-pity or pondering hibernation; relieved that I was alive. He told me how great he thought I was for holding it together. How great it was to be home and how much he loved me.

All I could say was, "Oh." What had I expected from this man? This was the man I married, a man of enduring character. It shouldn't have surprised me at all. Cancer had shown me something I had known all along but had thought might change. He was exactly the man I had married. Love and beauty are in the eye of the beholder, and to Tom, I was still Diane. What a blessing. So, life moved on and we moved on.

The reason Tom had come home from his own frantic schedule was so that we could take our son Tommy out for his tenth birthday. Turning ten in our house was a big deal. It was a tradition my parents had started when I was a kid. As the birthday kid, you were able to pick the restaurant, the conversation, and the entertainment for your birthday evening. These requests had to be within reason of course. So, I decided to put on my wig for the festivities. I had settled on a fine wig, but it was still a wig. I wasn't thrilled with it. I knew "my" hair didn't flip that way. "My" hair didn't have those highlights. "My" hair was nothing like this helmet I was wearing—but it would do the job.

I know people spend a lot of time trying to make these pieces look great. (And, just for the record, Cher's hairdresser is amazing.) But for us cancer patients, we know when we look in the mirror there's no hair underneath. No eyelashes. No brows. We know it's a polite thing we do for everyone else. It helps everyone to stay in their comfort zone. Fake hair is reassuring to those who want to believe that everything is all right. Sometimes we can even fool ourselves into thinking we are passing for normal. Most times, we just know you feel better.

Well, back to the special occasion of the birthday and my getting myself and my hair ready. My husband said we would take the Camaro. Now, this car was only for special occasions. It had a blankie and had been given gentle strokes and loving glances. This car had endless stories about it. However, key to my current predicament was that this car was a convertible. Tom didn't take this car out for any old reason. It had to be a big deal. As I imagined sitting in the seat of this car, my mind raced to my hair. All I could think of was my hair blowing off, sailing through the air like some animal that we had hit and looking like road kill lying on the shoulder. There I would be sitting with my scalp glistening in the sun. I would be the guilty party, the killer of the wig. I gathered myself, gave an extra tug downward, and headed down the stairs. As I came to the railing and peered down the stairs for our outing, I know Tom could tell I was uneasy. I shared with him the scene of what had just played out in my mind. His eyes crinkled, and we laughed about my wig hair blowing in the wind. At least if my hair went flying, we both had prepared ourselves for it.

Tom called for Tommy, and we headed to The Stonehouse. This is one of our favorite restaurants and was Tommy's choice. The ride over was uneventful, and my hair stayed where it was supposed to. We had a fabulous meal, as always. I don't remember pulling on the helmet of hair too much. Of course acquaintances commented on how "great" I looked and then moved on to the birthday boy. Dinner had gone off without a hitch and we were off to see *Star Wars* at the show. Two separate destinations with hair still intact. My husband and son covered me with compliments during the entire outing. I knew they were trying to make me feel good about the wig. I also knew my husband could sense my awkwardness with this new hair. I knew he was trying to read through any little gesture I made. I kept my gestures to a minimum.

We had a wonderful time. We all enjoyed the ride home and were satisfied with the success of Tommy's tenth birthday. Once we were alone at home, my husband jokingly told me I was going to have to learn to move my head with my hair. I asked if it was that obvious. "Only to me," he said. He asked me how I liked the wig. I thought for a minute and then it struck me—I hated the wig. It wasn't me. I felt like I had a giant suction cup on my head. I was stiff, and that wasn't me. I wasn't stiff. Tom said he didn't care if I wore the wig or not. He said he wasn't in love with my hair. He was happy if I was happy. He looked me straight in the eye and said he *really* didn't care about my hair. Wow. I sure love that guy! Decision made. Wigs were not for me. Hats would be my choice of covering. I felt they would provide a more comfortable distraction and a sense of security. So ladies, cut yourself some slack. Hair really is overrated in the big picture. The loss is strictly temporary.

The next big hair test came with my children. It was fall now and back-to-school time. This meant it was time to meet the teachers. Somehow I was sensing my son was not going to appear at school with me in a hat. After all, by this time I had accumulated a colorful variety of hats in my collection since so many friends found it a challenge to find me the latest and greatest hat. I should've known to clear it with my son. The younger children didn't seem to dwell on the lack of hair, and my oldest daughter was willing to work with whatever choice I made. Tommy Jr., on the other hand, requested that I wear hair for his teachers. It made me laugh.

Obviously, I needed to fit in as a normal mom. I needed to have hair. So on went the hair. I could deal with the awkwardness of the wig for a few hours of teacher meet and greet. I'm sure he figured if I could get through his birthday with hair intact, I certainly could make it through meet-the-teacher night. I cherish this memory because kids will let you know where they're at. "Like hey, I definitely need you to blend with the other parents tonight." So, I put on the dreaded wig, and after spending a fair amount of effort to look my best, I came out in all my glory for my son to inspect. He tilted his head to one side, and to my surprise he said, "Mom, no, you can go put your hat back on." *What?* I thought. After all that tugging and primping, I had been summarily dismissed by a ten-year-old. Obviously, the wig fell short of expectations and the hat would do. It seemed that the new normal of Mom was with no hair and a hat. Wow, totally accepted! This feeling warmed my heart. These were the only two times the wig ever saw daylight.

Chapter Twenty-Two

MORE TREATMENT

The months passed slowly by as I underwent my chemo treatments. My life had taken on this new pattern. My family and friends were all focused on helping me to get through this process. My back deck became HGTV's staging area for flowers, and I tried to keep my schedule as normal as possible. I did miss some work. I had many opportunities to take short jaunts out in the real world while I was traveling for treatment. People would see me and give me that knowing look or quickly look away. Mostly, it exposed me to others who were in the same or similar situations. The telltale sign of cancer, my hat, was obvious for everyone to see.

One of the most rewarding things about this time was that I often found myself mentoring complete strangers, telling them how I was getting through this episode in my life and sharing my faith. I wanted to give them hope to continue to move through the tunnel the same way others had encouraged me. I would emphasize to them and myself that I would get through this and so would they, and we couldn't focus on anything else. There was no point in focusing on anything else! These encounters were as much of an encouragement to me as I hope I was to them.

By the end of chemo, I was weaker than when I started, but I made it. I had gotten through that section of the cancer tunnel. After leaving my last treatment of poison, I felt my life starting a rewind. If I could have done one of my daughter's handsprings I would have. (Of course, that wasn't an option even before the chemo.) It was on to radiation. Nurses told me this would be more time consuming but less physically consuming. So they said! I'd see.

Chapter Twenty-Three

RADIATION

*R*adiation was the next section of the cancer tunnel. All things happen for a reason. We hear this said over and over. Most times we nod like we know, like we might even have a clue about the reason. But, I truly believe this. I didn't have a hint of why I was in this and going through this at this point in my life. Radiation, my next step, would help me to figure it out. The next six weeks revealed how it wasn't about me at all. The focus became someone else. Someone I'd never met before.

First of all, radiation doesn't leave you sickened like chemo does. That was true. Most of your body is blocked off from the effects because it's very focused. Soon I chose to attend some of these appointments on my own. I used the time to gather my thoughts and pray. It was a quiet time there and back. I treasured these times when I was left alone with my prayers and my God. Again, I felt Him. His Word worked through my mind and lifted my thoughts. Not always thoughts of this world but of the glory of the next. It gave me new perspective on all the time I had spent on things that didn't really matter. I got a lot out of those drives by myself, and it prepared me for my future meeting with an unknown woman named Phyllis. My daily visits had become mundane. I got up, went to my part- time job, drove sixty miles, went to a ten-minute radiation treatment, drove back, went home, and then went to bed. The next day I did it all over again. This part of my life was just following the doctor's orders.

I thought six weeks sounded like an unending length of time. All I had to do was to take care of myself. I just wanted it to hurry by so I could get on to the next phase.

Chapter Twenty-Four

HAROLD & PHYLLIS

Two weeks into radiation, I found myself sitting in a room full of cancer patients. I was waiting to go into treatment, when I noticed a woman sitting across from me who looked like she needed a hug. Yeah well, we all need a hug. I don't believe in coincidences, but I do believe in divine appointments. You know, the whole blooming where you are planted thing ... but giving a stranger a hug wasn't one of the opportunities I usually look for. Still, the urge to go over and give this woman a hug was powerful. She looked frail and ready to depart this world at any minute. This "hug" thought was completely outside of my comfort zone, but I couldn't shake the overwhelming prompting I was feeling. What to do? What else could I do? I decided to be obedient to this silent command.

I believe that when you are feeling really close to God, you are more attentive to His direction, but I wasn't sure if this was one of those times. My life during radiation had been pretty much me and God in the car for sixty minutes there and sixty minutes back. This seemed like direct orders from Him. I felt the need to follow this prompting, hoping it really was His idea. So, I went in obedience.

"Hi … you look like you could use a hug today." She looked up and smiled. Her face beamed warmly, and I took it as approval for my offer. I leaned down and gave the warmest hug I could to this complete stranger. A man seated nearby, who I assumed was her husband, gave me a strange look. I told them my name and where I was from. She told me their names and where they were from. We proceeded to make small talk. I laid out details about myself, and they responded with information about themselves. Soon, we were talking about our cancers. I soon found she had little to hope for in her cancer journey. I explained how I, on the other hand, had a lot to hope for. I felt a little uncomfortable that her situation was so dire, and the worst part of it all was that they had no one to nurture them through this experience. Our encounter was very brief. Just as quickly as it started, it was over. I thought about them all the way home.

The next treatment, I found myself alone again except for Phyllis, my hug friend. We soon struck up a conversation. It felt like we had known each other forever. She and her husband told me how they pretty much kept to themselves. It didn't seem from our conversation that they had much going on, other than cancer. It also seemed like they didn't have much in the way of finances either. There was no involved family. They lived alone in an apartment building. They didn't have much to say about their neighbors. No pets. There were just the two of them.

My eyes consumed them as we talked. I took in all the details of their physical presence in the waiting room. Her body looked frail and tattered. She really was a sight to behold. Again, the prompting was there for me to intervene. Oh great, how was I going to do that? *Shopping!* Yes, shopping popped into my head. Not for me, but for her. On the way home I asked God to tell me what my purpose was in this. Phyllis looked as if she could use a new robe and slippers. I couldn't believe the direction was about clothing, but hey, I can't explain why God does anything He does. So I went out and purchased a soft pink robe and slippers. I presented these gifts to her at our next meeting. Phyllis and Harold seemed overwhelmed that I had identified a need and filled it. Immediately they began to open up more to me. Soon I found them arriving early to spend time with me. Harold said he felt as if I were an angel sent to them. Wow, no one had ever accused me of that before. But this relationship continued, and I tried to follow my heart because I had no idea what my purpose was in this series of events.

I told my husband about this couple, and he agreed to even drive down to have dinner with Phyllis and Harold. Our relationship began to expand outside of the chemo treatments. It wasn't a smooth relationship. I really only barely knew these people. Cancer had been the initial cause of our contact, but I believed there was another reason yet to be revealed. My husband wasn't quite sure where this was all going and wondered what we could possibly do for these people. All I knew was the Lord was leading, and I was following. Harold and Phyllis had no family, few friends, and no faith to lean on. They were very much alone. I knew that they appreciated my attention, and I knew that they wanted to share themselves with me. Tom was supportive and attended the events I asked him to.

My meetings with Phyllis and Harold went on for four weeks, until one of my last visits when I arrived to see that they were noticeably absent. I asked the nurse, "Where are they?" She informed me that Phyllis had taken a turn for the worse and was in the hospital. After treatment, I immediately headed for the hospital. There sat Harold. Phyllis was lying in bed looking weak and frail. She was failing. Harold was stoically watching over her.

I walked in and asked him what had happened. Harold explained that she had developed a sudden case of pneumonia, and I sensed in his spirit that he was preparing for Phyllis's eventual death. Phyllis could barely talk, but she squeezed my hand as I reached and held hers. I could see that she wanted to talk. Her eyes looked deeply into mine for the moments they stayed open. Her words were breathless and did not come easily. I felt God's urging to speak of Him to her. The salvation message was heavy on my heart. I needed confirmation. How was I going to do this with this elderly couple? I barely knew them, and maybe they would be offended. I knew I needed help with this. For now, I would have to leave the two of them. I couldn't stay any longer, and I needed to organize myself. I knew that wherever two or more are gathered in God's name, He will be there.

So, all the way home I thought of who would be my helper with this task. Okay, here comes the ironic part. It came to me. I knew who I had to get on this mission with me—one of my dearest friends. Funny, but her name is Phyllis. I called Phyllis and explained the situation. She listened quietly and then agreed it had to be done. Time was slipping away. The next day, Phyllis headed off with me to my radiation appointment. As quickly as I could, I went through my treatment. Phyllis and I then proceeded to the other Phyllis's location to lend any help or comfort we could.

We arrived at the hospital and headed directly to the room. The room was still. Now, the witnessing Phyllis pulls no punches. There's no grand performance but a gentle reasoning of the facts and how they play out for eternity, and she does all of this with love dripping off her words. I quickly made the introduction to Harold and then we took up our stations. I was on one side of the bed-ridden Phyllis, while my friend, Phyllis, was on the other side. We both leaned onto the hospital bed and shared God's love and grace. Occasionally I looked up at Harold and sensed that he was comforted and overjoyed that so much attention was being given to his wife, with nothing expected in return. She was nodding her head ever so slightly. Her hands held firmly on to Phyllis's and mine. We knew she understood. Just as sweetly as it started, it was over. She had chosen to give her heart to the Lord. It was one of the most blessed things I had ever witnessed. All three of us women had tears in our eyes and hearts at peace. Even Harold had tears streaming down his face. He found his voice and said, "Why would anyone take the time to care this much about someone they barely know?"

Cancer could not invade this holy place.

Not long after, I got the call. Phyllis had died. I knew it was coming. I rejoiced that Phyllis was in the arms of her Savior. I wasn't prepared for what else Harold had to say.

"Diane?"

"Yes, Harold."

"Would you come and give the service for Phyllis? I know she would like that."

"Harold, what about a pastor or a family member?" I said.

"No, there isn't anyone, and I know Phyllis would want it to be you."

"All right—when and where, and are you sure?"

Harold confirmed that he was sure, and then he supplied me with the details.

I'd never done a funeral service. I felt completely inadequate in this role, but again felt the nudge that my mission wasn't complete. Tom wasn't sure it was appropriate. We consulted our pastor. I explained to our pastor that they had no one else in their lives to do it. Our pastor told us that a funeral didn't require an expert. Tom agreed to attend with me and help however he could.

The funeral was sparsely attended. A few neighbors from their apartment complex had shown up. The funeral director and Tom and I rounded out the group. I couldn't help thinking that this is where life could end up for some: a handful of neighbors and strangers paying their last respects.

Things got underway very quickly. There was no big procession of guests to wade through and no elaborate ceremony to dictate the pace. I moved to the front and began my service for Phyllis. I described how I had come to know Phyllis and her husband. I talked about our few engagements together and how we had connected in such a short period of time. I explained how she and Harold had become an integral part of my cancer treatment routine. Most importantly, I ended with the message I believe I had been divinely appointed to deliver to Phyllis and Harold, the salvation message. I poured as much love as I could into those words and then, just as quickly it was over.

After the service, an elderly woman came up to Tom and me and introduced herself. She was one of Phyllis's neighbors. She had been praying for Phyllis for many years. She had often tried to make inroads into the closed life of Harold and Phyllis to no avail. She had invited them to her church, brought treats over, and tried to be as friendly as a person could be. Still, all her efforts had fallen short of the goal. She thanked me for being an answer to prayer. I looked at Tom and he looked at me. They were powerful words for us. Another stranger had just confirmed that we had been used in the most profound way possible. I felt at peace that my mission had been completed. The salvation message had been given, and Phyllis had received it.

I honestly have to say I don't know whether Harold ever took that step. I hope he did. I did hear from his estranged daughter that he had passed not long after Phyllis. I prayed that my mission had been accomplished and that I had clearly discerned the Lord's direction in this event.

Chapter Twenty-Five

THE HOLIDAYS

oon enough the holidays were upon me. I finished radiation on a Wednesday ... the day before Thanksgiving. I was so grateful to be able to be done for the holidays. I knew I wouldn't be 100 percent for the festivities, but I was one step closer to the finish line. Also, having radiation out of my schedule freed me up to participate in the traditional family activities.

Fortunately for me, my mother had a Thanksgiving dinner that I only had to show up for. I knew there would be plenty of everything, and I could just relax and enjoy the celebration. All of my siblings would be there. It would give me an opportunity to visit with everyone all in one shot, because I honestly didn't know if I had the energy to do more than that. Treatment had left me physically and emotionally exhausted.

As my family and I arrived at my parents' house, we were greeted with happy faces and concerned hugs. I glanced around and took in the warmth of it all. There's nothing like the smell of your mother's kitchen—especially on Thanksgiving. The table was covered with every kind of delicious holiday fare. My sisters and my brother and his family had outdone themselves with the preparations. I'm sure my family was eyeing all the home-cooked delicacies.

After many questions and navigating through the waters of cancer treatment, we all found our seats around the table. A prayer was offered, and it held great meaning for me. I can't speak for everyone else, but I do believe we all were far more aware of our blessings this Thanksgiving. Life is a fragile, precious gift.

Before we all started passing the plates, I had noticed my sister, Linda, had left the room. I wondered what she was up to. Before long, in she came with a plate bearing a separate, miniature turkey. In celebration of my completion of this latest stage of treatment, my sister felt it was appropriate to present me with my own personal Thanksgiving Turkey: a Cornish hen. We all laughed, and the twinkle in Linda's eye was obvious. She had found a special, funny way to single me out and lighten the mood. I loved it!

I enjoyed Thanksgiving and one of the best Christmas experiences of my life. I knew everyone had pictured the possibility of those holidays coming with me not there. I was truly focused on the joy of being present. I didn't know what the future would hold, but I knew we were all more mindful of the true spirit of the season. I believe we were all more thankful than in the years past.

Chapter Twenty-Six

LIFE GOES ON

As always, it doesn't matter what is going on with you personally because life goes on. It must.

I didn't have the distraction of the holidays any longer, so I spent time running through my mind what I had just been through in these past several months. This cancer experience had taken me to the edge of death. My body had been filled with poison and maximum levels of radiation. My strength and will had been stretched to the point of never returning to normal. Now, all of a sudden, I had been freed to resume life. How do you do that? The doctors and nurses didn't give me a pamphlet or anything outlining the resumption of life. I felt like a wet noodle. Where do I go to begin to find normal? I had the one comforting thought that the cancer in me was now dead, but how did I get back to Diane strength? I didn't feel like myself. I was functioning and that's about it. My family was buzzing about and their lives were going at the same speed, but I felt stuck in Jell-O. What would it take to get back up to the normal speed of life? I knew in my soul that I was sick and tired of feeling sick and tired. I didn't want the only time of the day that sounded appealing to be bedtime, but what should I do? I didn't have a plan, but I knew in my heart this couldn't last. This would have to be another beginning of life after cancer. How was I going to start? I had no ideas.

January came, and I was still in a pit. What could I do? Was I depressed? No, but I wasn't up. I knew I needed some kind of movement. Rolling over on the couch didn't count anymore. I had been involved in regular exercise in the past, so it came to me that this would be one of the best ways to spark my energy. That was where I decided to start—the good ole' YMCA.

The YMCA was going to be a scheduling nightmare around my family's already busy days. Whatever ... I needed to do this. I knew it was important. I knew I had to make it as crucial as a daily vitamin. God hadn't spared me so I could lie on the couch and watch the sun rise and set while my family went on living and I watched. So, I decided every chance I had, I would pull on my cancer hat and head off to recover my health. YMCA here I come!

As I first walked through the door of the YMCA, I wondered if people would notice my cancer stamp: no hair. No one said anything or tried to grab my hat like kids do when they suspect something is up. I carefully proceeded to the treadmill. I looked at the settings intently and couldn't find the "after cancer, stuck in Jell-O" setting, so I set the dial to the slooooowest of slow speeds! At first, I thought someone would be taping this for *America's Funniest Home Videos*, because I felt so obviously awkward, but I didn't see any hidden cameras anywhere so I stepped aboard. I turned on the treadmill. I was able to go a whole three minutes. That's right—a whole three minutes. My heart sank. Three minutes sounded ridiculous. I was completely exhausted and left the Y in tears. I had just given "weak" a whole new bottom level.

I returned home wondering what kind of drugs or verbal abuse I was going to have to put myself through to go back to the Y and endure the humiliation all over again. Cancer had stripped me of my hair and my energy. It had tried to kill me. Now I had to decide if I would let myself settle into that life of weakness.

The next morning, I knew I couldn't quit before even starting. Every inch of me was crying "no," but I knew I had to persevere. I got in my car and returned to the Y and the torturous treadmill. By the end of the week I was up to ten minutes. Woohoo, double digits. I persevered. Isn't that what we are called to do? "Can I get an Amen?" "Amen."

As I continued to go to the Y, I started to feel comfortable with the other clients. I saw the same two women over and over. They looked like they knew what they were doing. They looked great. You know that healthy "I-go-to-the-Y" look! I was hoping they wouldn't notice my pathetic attempt at endurance. I kept my hat low and my head focused.

When Easter arrived, I decided to display my new Easter bonnet: a short covering of dark curls. This new cancer style was easy to maintain, and others complimented me on the look. Apparently it agreed with me or people were just relieved to see hair on my head. I decided to leave my baseball cap home as I headed out for the Y.

The same two women took an interest in me and cheered me on. Debbie and Denise were at the Y daily, and they talked as we walked. They shared about themselves and their routine, and I shared about myself and why I was there. They poured their words of encouragement into me, and those supportive words are stamped on my heart forever. Denise encouraged me to take a weight course and master how to improve my well-being. She told me this would help me build my body strength back. I truly believe their presence was integral to my motivation and divinely appointed. I admired their abilities and wanted their health for myself. I wanted to know what that felt like to be strong again. Total health had become like a faded memory. The only person who could bring it back was me. I knew the scars from my battle were still left to be dealt with, but I could start on the inside and work my way out.

Over time I noticed my grocery bags were getting lighter. I was making progress. Day by day the effort got easier. Now it was spring, and I took myself outside. Where I live you don't waste one good weather day because you never know when the snow will hit again. I started to feel healthier. I was walking, then race walking, and eventually ended up running on the street. The treadmill and I had an amicable breakup once the weather turned nice. He knew he was just the transition guy.

Debbie told me she was going to hold me accountable to continue to exercise outside. She made a point of showing up at my place of work to walk with me. I was so grateful. This lasted for several months, and I know having her there for accountability is what kept me going on my path to revival. As my progress continued, my life started to feel normal—even better than normal. My family wasn't running circles around me. I could keep up. My daily exercise was my daily medicine. It had brought me from the brink of exhaustion and despair. Spring turned into summer, summer into fall, and fall into winter. My endurance continued to increase, and I felt good.

The weather dictated that I make my amends with the treadmill. I approached reluctantly, but I was welcomed back with open arms. What a softie!

I ran almost daily all through the winter, and a five-mile run became easy. The same two gals were there consistently. I overheard their conversations of competition and marathons. Wow, they were better than I had even imagined. They were real runners. Then on one of my typical visits to the YMCA, a pivotal question came my way from the two of them.

"Have you ever thought of competing in a race?" Debbie asked.

"Uhhhhh … I'm not competitive." I replied

"You don't have to be," she said. "It's just fun to be out there with other runners."

"Really? I thought you guys were a special breed." I smiled.

"No, we just keep going." Debbie said.

"Yeah, right … ha ha … just keep going. Funny."

Could I run a marathon? Nooo … well, maybe. It struck me funny that they had gone right to the subject of a marathon, since this had been a previous college goal of mine never fulfilled. How funny to have it resurface at this odd time.

Well, they said I could and they should know. They were probably just being nice. You know, like awww … let's try to build her up. The question came again. Now, these girls knew about my cancer. How could they expect me to run a marathon? They didn't seem concerned about that at all. What if I failed? What if people thought I was crazy? What if, what if, what if. What if I succeeded?

Soon the idea was making itself comfortable in my brain. I was really entertaining the idea. My runs took on a new momentum. With each step, I considered the thought of entering a race. There was a 5K that was being offered through the Y. I'd sign up for that. What could it hurt? I was past the point of worrying about embarrassment. Walking around as a bald woman takes the sting out of being stared at.

I pressed forward. This would be my first real test as a runner, more importantly, as a survivor. I entered. I ran. I finished in the middle—but I finished. It was true … you didn't need to be an Olympian to run a race. It felt great. Not physically great, but "I-did-it" great. Great … like I could do this!

My family was happy for my accomplishments. Some people did think I was crazy. Funny how it is the people you don't expect to doubt you, that do. It is no wonder why we spend so much of our lives trying to explain ourselves. But once again, I knew this was something I had to do, for me. For anyone who was watching me who might get their own diagnosis. For those who thought I should sit down and rock the rest of my life away. For my family who needed to know I was okay. I know they were relieved: relieved that I appeared strong, relieved that the focus was slowly drifting away from cancer, relieved that life was taking on a new normal. A healthy normal! Cancer was losing its grip on my time, but I knew I still had a ways to go in my spirit.

It was my spirit that responded when I was challenged again. Debbie suggested training for the Chicago Marathon. "I mean if you're running six miles you can surely do twenty-six." Now that seemed like a big difference to me, but Debbie and Denise shrugged it off like "how silly."At first I had my usual "no-way" reaction. Debbie pressed harder. My spirit quickened at the thought, and I knew I had to prove to myself that I could do it. I weighed all the factors and decided I was in. The training began. Life continued at its usual pace, only now I had added a twenty-six-mile marathon to the to-do list. Yeah, no biggie, right? I could maybe do this. Yeah!

So that spring and summer I diligently trained for the big day. The training was consistent and intense. Sometimes, time management was an issue. I should've seen that coming. I mean, I'd just been through cancer, a huge time commitment. A marathon would be training every day. Also, where do you squeeze a ten-mile run in? Before grocery shopping, after the dog groomer? How about once everyone is in bed? Nope, you've got to have cooperation. Once again, my family rose to the challenge. They cheered me on without complaint. I believe they were encouraged that they were witnessing me transform from a weak, tired mom into a motivated, healthy mom. Their support was astounding.

Surprisingly, I never felt like I couldn't do this. I did wonder how I would add the miles I needed to reach twenty-six miles. But, each time, I amazed myself by being able to add the two I needed. I attribute this to my rigid training schedule. I had bought the book *The Complete Woman's Guide to Running,* and I was sticking to it. I mean, this woman wrote a book about the subject. She must be legit.

Some people thought my goals were ridiculous. Others were enthusiastic. A few thought it was a desperate cry for attention. All I can say is think of the movie *Forrest Gump* when Forrest runs back and forth across the country, over and over, to escape the thoughts of the woman he loves. Well, I needed to escape cancer once and for all. I now needed to know that I could endure twenty-six miles of physical agony that only a healthy person could endure. I wanted to do more than just survive. I wanted to live and dream and hope that I might be able to bless others with my story.

I found through training that my whole inner being was transformed. My sluggish attitude was replaced by a euphoric new lease on life! The whole process of getting fit and healthy was contagious. My family jumped on the healthy train and rode with me through the process. I finally understood what it meant to take care of yourself so that you could take care of others. I realized that I had more staying power. I felt good when called upon, not frustrated and tired. It was true that being caring to yourself is the responsible thing to do.

The date was set. Chicago, here I come.

Before I ran in Chicago, I continued to enter some of our local races. I used them as training runs. At every race I would run alongside people and ask them questions: How did you get started running? How do you keep going when your body aches? Why do you keep running? Do you want to win or is it just for fun? Fortunately, no one tripped me to shut me up. They were all anxious to share their stories and their advice. They all had their own unique stories and tricks of the trade. I found it all fascinating and encouraging.

Chapter Twenty-Seven

MACKINAC ISLAND RACE

*T*here was one race that proved to be very special for me. It was the Eight-Mile Mackinac Island Race. This race is about 150 miles from my home. It was scheduled in the fall and that would put it about one month prior to Chicago. It sounded like the perfect little getaway with my family. It would be great practice training for Chicago. Besides, who wouldn't love to run around Mackinac Island? It was one of the gems of the Upper Peninsula of Michigan. My family loved the idea and soon it was race day.

My family and I boarded the ferry for the island. As we glided through the cool blue waves of Lake Huron in the giant hovercraft, my mind settled on how this race might truly make me feel like a real competitor. I had become confident in my new stamina. I had developed a decent stride and definitely improved my speed. I actually was getting that competitive bug. Not the Olympic competitive bug, but the "hey-Diane-not-bad" bug.

We landed on the island where time had been stopped. No cars, just horses. There were cute Victorian shops and tons of runners. I quickly headed to the starting point, and my family wished me well. I stood there shaking out with the best of them. I didn't feel like people were staring at me. I was excited. You could feel the anticipation. I felt like a runner.

Pop! ... went the gun, and we were off. Soon all the people running closest to me became my new best friends. We were all excitedly talking about the race, the day, and running in general. As the miles wore on, some of my new friends quickly pulled ahead, some fell behind. I was maintaining my pace, the middle. Three miles into the race, I noticed a new woman running alongside of me. She looked to be about my age, and she immediately began to talk. I welcomed the conversation. Talking always made the distance seem shorter to me.

Within a few short minutes she began to tell me that she had just been diagnosed with breast cancer. This would be her final run before radical surgery and treatment. She was facing surgery and a treatment regimen far more drastic than what I had just been through. I listened as she poured out the details of cancer's arrival in her life. I almost stopped with the shock of it all, but one foot kept moving in front of the other. I don't know how long it took, but when she got to the end of her story, I offered up mine. I went through my own discovery, anger, surgery, treatment, recovery, and search for renewal. Humbly, I offered my encouragement. We shared glances of knowing. Knowing what only another human being can know who's heard those words: You have cancer.

Everything else about the day drifted away. The beautiful island, my finishing time, my competitive spirit all replaced. It was all replaced by the making of a bond that would follow me into every situation for the rest of my life, the bond of cancer.

I knew I was in the middle of another divine appointment. I knew what the real point of this race day was. We finished the race together, praying together, arm in arm, tears streaming down our faces, thanking God for bringing us together. It was the most powerful race I had run. I had been blessed. I had been used to help someone else carry their burden and another stitch had gone into the repair of my spirit. It was proof again that God will use us in the most powerful ways if only we will be open and willing.

This race confirmed my conviction to press on to my goal. My running was not just for my physical healing. It had become my spiritual and emotional healing as well. I was so truly thankful. I had just made another "breast friend."

One month until Chicago.

Chapter Twenty-Eight

OUT OF NOWHERE

*P*olitical life? As I mentioned previously, my husband was a logger. In a situation that I can only describe as another divine intervention, my husband was thrust into the political arena. Now, at this point in my life, politics was way down on the "have-to-do" list. However, the timber industry was going through its own trauma, and Tom felt compelled to get involved. His grassroots involvement produced results. How he was able to focus on anything was beyond me, but he did. The legislation in our state was changed. Looking back, I know this legislation was a good diversion from always worrying about me.

Now, I'm going to let you in on a secret. As a private citizen, if you are ever able to move government legislatively, expect someone to ask you if you've ever thought of running for office. Tom had always been aware and attentive to politics, but until this experience, had little thought of running for office. He liked being a logger! I certainly never thought of politics. Who would?!

It wasn't long before the question came. They wanted Tom to consider running as a state representative. It would be a total gamble on our future. Personally, I was not looking to play the percentages on anything again. Tom wasn't sure he could do it along with everything else that was already going on in our lives. It would be a huge commitment and would be another financial hurdle. We were undecided, and that was where we would leave it.

Tom and I were invited out to an all-expense-paid special award presentation. This was a national award presented by The American Loggers Council. Tom would be receiving this special annual award for his efforts in the logging industry. This ceremony was right before I was scheduled to run in my marathon. Tom knew how important it was for me to get to Chicago for the race. He knew the training I had devoted to my quest. I knew the effort he had put forth to help his industry. I knew it would be wonderful for him to be recognized for his work. So, we decided we would go to the prepaid ceremony in Lake Tahoe, California, then dash off to Chicago for the race. It would be a tight schedule, but we committed to do it. Traveling allowed us to talk even more about the possibility of political life. How would we do it? Tom wasn't sure he even could do it. He was already so busy with the business. We headed to the event with a lot of unanswered questions.

Tom's acceptance speech was fabulous, and it was the first time I heard Tom mention publicly that he was considering running for political office. I had the strangest feeling that after, hopefully, completing my marathon, I was going to transition into a political marathon. I couldn't focus on this right now. I had to think about my race.

We arrived in Reno at 5 a.m. for our flight to Chicago. It was necessary for us to get to the airport hours before our flight due to the post-9/11 security. We didn't arrive in Chicago until 5:00 p.m. We took a taxi to the hotel and met up with our kids and friends. They were our pastor and his wife, Diane from home. Their daughter from St. Louis was there to run the marathon too.

They had come to cheer the two of us on. Diane had completely outfitted our rooms with banners and various paraphernalia, all to signify her love and pride in our endeavor. It was a comfort for my nerves to see everyone and our rooms.

My husband and children were bouncy with excitement. We had to settle down and get some sleep. As we unpacked, the phone began to ring with calls from well-wishers. My brother, who had run the Boston Marathon, called and shared his encouragement and knowing excitement. My mother called with love and never-ending parental concern and good-luck wishes. Friends called with their cheers. There was no way I was going to be able to calm my mind.

I ate my carb overload meal at 9 p.m. I needed to go to bed. I couldn't sleep. I tried, but all I could think was if I did, how I might sleep through the start time.

Eventually, my eyes closed. The next thing I knew, I was waking to my alarm and grabbing my energy-packed breakfast. The whole room was abuzz with activity. Each of us was grabbing our stuff and snacks and out we stumbled. Off we all went to the race site. We soon were caught up in the crowds which were all moving in the same direction. I had to get into the flow of the runners, and my family and friends had to get into the flow of those waiting by alphabet to greet the finishers.

Race morning was an experience. Forty-five thousand runners were lined up by times. This mass of humanity was shaking limbs, smiling knowingly at each other, and waiting for the gun to go off. Soon we were one large parade making our way through the race route. The whole city had come out to celebrate our attempt at greatness. There was entertainment and happy spirits the whole way. People I didn't even know were handing out water, bananas, and conversation. People were sharing and cheering and encouraging. At twenty miles, I had a man come alongside me and tell me this was just the start of a typical six-mile training day. Wow just six more miles. It helped me for three miles, and after that the strain started to weigh on me again. The last three miles took me forty-five minutes.

I was wondering if this was going to end the way I wanted it to. All those names I had written on my shirt and those who had written themselves on my heart kept me going. All those cancer relationships had brought me to this point and were now pushing me forward. One foot kept going in front of the other, not quickly but consistently. Soon the finish line was in front of me. Could it be? It was. I could feel the emotions welling up inside. As my body crossed the finish I was embraced, congratulated, and wrapped in love—and a medal was hung around my neck. Tears streamed down my face and sobs wracked my body. I had done it. We had done it. It was finished. Looking back, I think the medal hanger had the best job of the whole race. That person was the recipient of all the relief and gratitude of a race won.

Quickly, I headed for my family. People couldn't wait for you at the finish line, so I had to go find them. It was all very organized by name and place. I'm sure it would have been a much easier task if I hadn't been trying to do it with tears in my eyes. I shouldn't say in my eyes, because they weren't staying; they were flowing uncontrollably down my face. I'm sure I was a sight. Every fiber of me was aching and screaming for joy all at the same time.

As I approached my designated location, I was embraced once more and surrounded in my family's and friends' love. It was a sense of affirmation I would never forget. They all congratulated me, and we all talked at once. They were so proud I had done it. I know they were happy it was over, and so was I. In my mind I had run cancer into twenty-six miles of pavement. I had run it out of my life. I had run it out of my family's life. It was time to close the book on cancer and start writing, "the rest of my story."

Chapter Twenty-Nine

CAMPAIGN 2002

*T*hat whole next year took all of our energy. Tom and I entered an endeavor we had little knowledge of. Tom and I had discussed it and decided he would put all his energy into running for state rep for our district. We combined this with my cancer checkups, and I kept running and working to maintain my new healthy lifestyle. Life was chugging along.

Our family's schedule began a new rhythm. Not that campaign life is normal, but it was milder than logging so it became the new normal. I was once again enjoying raising my family, working out at the Y, going for my six- month checkups at Mayo, humming along.

At one of my checkups, I received one of the finest prescriptions ever from a doctor. I had explained to my doctor that I was having some anxiety, mood swings, and at times overall dislike of myself. She reminded me that I was taking Tamoxifen, and that this particular drug acts like a pseudo-estrogen and as a result there really wasn't any hormone therapy I could take to relieve symptoms. My doctor looked straight at me and very pointedly asked, "Do you drink?" I clarified that she was referring to alcohol, and then I replied, "No, not really." "Well, the health benefits of red wine can have the calming effect that you could benefit from," she said. What? Did I just hear my doctor tell me to drink? The look on my face must have made clear what I was thinking. She reassured me that this was not a license to drink. She limited the prescription to an occasional four-ounce glass with dinner. This was not medical advice. This was advice from a woman I had come to regard as a confidant and a breast friend.

At this same appointment, we discussed the possibility of restoring some of my visual femininity. No, it wasn't possible to erase all the scars, but there were options for some restoration. Not that concave isn't unique and special (I hope you are sensing my sarcasm here), but for me it didn't quite fill out the turtleneck like I wanted. There really isn't anything to compete with a decent breast. If both breasts had been removed, then there definitely would have been a certain symmetry going on, but only one man was left standing. I wanted to eliminate the daily look in the mirror at my loss. She informed me that Mayo had a wonderful reconstruction surgeon. He would be hard to get in to see, but he was definitely worth the wait. Boy I'd heard that before, but I trusted this woman. She said she would make the initial contact and keep me posted.

I returned home thinking about this reconstruction when another "breast friend" came into my life. Tom and I were sitting in the local bagel shop when the owners came over to chat. Tom struck up a conversation with the husband, and I did likewise with his wife, Jean. Small talk turned into realizing that we shared the bond of surviving breast cancer. Breast cancer tears down any walls of pretense and immediately pushes your discussion to a very personal level. Next thing I knew, I was being pulled into the bathroom to examine a fully fledged reconstruction. I was in awe and encouraged. If there was any chance I could have even close to the result I was looking at, I was ready to sign up. Jean was ecstatic to show the results that could be achieved. She immediately took up her cheerleading pom-poms and exploded with encouragement. I was giddy with questions, and we chatted like schoolgirls who had found our own secret.

When Jean and I emerged from the bathroom, I could see the questioning look on my husband's face. He had to be wondering what had transpired in the last twenty minutes that had us laughing and hugging like we'd known each other since grade school.

Once Tom and I were in the car, I explained the whole event. He smiled knowing I had just made another "breast friend." Someone who was uniquely qualified to deliver just the right advice and confirmation of the decision I had made to go ahead with my own reconstruction. I couldn't wait to start the process (although it ended up taking six months to get an appointment). I knew Jean and I had just started a journey together. Later, I would find out how profoundly she would impact me and my family. I cherish her and our friendship to this day.

Another appointment that I didn't sign up for came calling. My comrade-in-arms, the woman who had shaved my head and wiped my tears, called to tell me she had been diagnosed with breast cancer. I was traveling alone when the call came. "Diane, I have some bad news." Shock shook me to the core as she described her diagnosis. I couldn't believe it. It was like hearing it for myself all over again. I knew from that moment on I would hear it over and over out of a variety of sources. Also, how could I be the friend that she had been for me? She was amazing, the one friend that everyone needs. The one who is always checking on you and making you feel like you're the only thing on her list. I would shoot for half of amazing and hope she didn't notice the other half.

Tom came with me to the appointment. At the consult, the doctor, the wonderful reconstruction surgeon Dr. T, came in with his nurse, another Phyllis, and a student colleague. I know, crazy. What are the chances, but it's true. So there I was with my husband, two other men, and Phyllis number three, trying to decide how my breasts should look. Breasts by committee. Instantly, I felt a connection with these two people. If he had been carrying a staff I would have sworn he could have parted the Red Sea. Phyllis would be with me every step of the way. She was with Dr. T from consult to completion. I didn't need anything parted, just put back. We went over all the options and settled on an expander that would be placed under the chest wall muscle and would stretch it and the skin which would allow for a future silicon implant. The skin and muscle would need to have basically a small hot-water bottle placed under it and have it filled every two weeks.

Well guess who got the pleasure of stretching me for the breast. My good friend Diane. She had been the one to shave my head and hold my hand, and she had always made herself available to me since the beginning of this whole cancer journey. Now I would ask her to go above and beyond the call of duty and hoped that she would let me put her into action again. I hope everyone who reads this has a friend like Diane. As I said before, she is a part of my soul. Also, if you're out there looking for a Diane, I should also tell you that she is an LPN. She knew all about sterile technique, and that is what I needed at my filling station. So for six months, every two weeks Diane came over for coffee and breast filling. We laughed at how life throws things at us that we could never have imagined ourselves doing. I tried not to hurt Diane when the skin and muscle that was being stretched started to burn with each filling. I questioned why I would choose this elective procedure. The skin had to be stretched larger than the breast would be in order to get a good result. Wow, the things you do for a nice-looking sweater.

Once the stretching of my skin and muscle was completed, I would have to wait another six months to let everything settle. The muscle needed to conform to the stretched position. If we didn't wait long enough the muscle could boomerang, and it would have all been for naught. Dr. T assured me that my patience would pay off. I trusted him, but my patience was wearing thin. I wanted to be done. He said no. I spent six more months working on the side that needed more TLC. The one side was a lovely summer fruit. The other side of my chest had a puny winterberry. That's as far as I'm going to go in the description of the predicament I was in. Use your imagination. Dr. T wanted the best possible results, and so did I. Another six months it would be.

It was finally here. Surgery would replace the expander and a silicone implant would go in. I was given a choice, and after tons of research, I was satisfied that all safety concerns had been resolved concerning the silicone. I liked the more natural feel of the silicone.

Once again, I woke up from surgery and thought one should not have to go through this much trauma for a decent pair of breasts. The pain was manageable, and I was hoping the scarring would be worth a full bra. One thing I had learned was I would have to wait for about a month to see what was left over after the swelling subsided. Another task accomplished on the road of reconstruction. Whatever the mirror revealed would have to do. Lucky for me … I liked what I saw.

Chapter Thirty

2006

*N*o one on the street would have guessed I had survived cancer. My life was full. My family was growing, kids were graduating, and we had built a new house … yada yada yada. I did a lot of entertaining now that my husband had taken on a political job. I had always loved to entertain, and Tom always felt confident that I could make a meal out of what was in the pantry. I loved to cook, and as a result, Tom never hesitated to ask colleagues or friends or both over for a meal.

Tom had asked me if I would be available to have some new guests for dinner one evening. They were a couple whom I had never met: Jan and Pete. Tom had met the husband and liked him very much. They were new in town. So, I know my husband figured it was time to get us girls together. I loved meeting new people, so I put on my hostess hat and got busy. They arrived, dinner went great. One of those dinners where you talk and talk and think to yourself, "we must be related or something." We had a lot in common except for her Southern accent. She was from Georgia and very honest and open. We clicked. I thought, *I'm going to be friends with her forever.* Sometimes you just know it. After three hours of camaraderie, we parted. I didn't know it then but she would play an integral part in my life. To be continued …

My hostess skills had survived cancer, and I was soon preparing for another dinner party. I looked forward to these occasions. Great new friends to make, great food to eat, and great conversation and dessert to finish an enjoyable evening. There would be four couples for this evening, but only one, Nikki and her husband, Tom, stayed late. The two Toms were having one of those brief conversations. (That's funny, because my husband is not known for his "brief" conversations.)

Nikki and I discussed our shared experience of breast cancer. We didn't see each other often, but we had that unbreakable bond of women who had survived cancer. We talked in detail about our trials and triumphs. Both of us had recovered some semblance of normalcy. I found myself telling her about the role my faith had played in my experience. I described how such a crisis had forced me to draw ever closer to my God, and that a trial so taxing had strengthened my dependence on Him. I explained to Nikki how I couldn't compare being in the arms of God to anything else. I remember specifically saying to her, "Sometimes I almost wish that a difficult time would come so that I could feel that again." It wasn't that I wanted cancer again, but I had discovered how quickly we move on when the trial has passed. I had found comfort in God's arms and there was nothing better.

The two Toms had ended their discussion, and Nikki and I parted. It had been another pleasant evening. Tom and I headed up to bed. Suddenly, I stopped on the steps, and that little speech I had shared with Nikki ran through my head. I knew something was up. I had that overwhelming feeling that I would be tested again, and that what I had just shared with Nikki had been a reminder for me, spoken through me.

Chapter Thirty-One

CANCER'S RETURN

*T*wo weeks later I was in the shower and felt a lump on the left side of my left breast. I didn't panic. I once again told myself this was a nonissue. I know. How could anyone who had just been through what I had been through think that? I have no idea. My guess is … it just didn't seem possible. How could it be anything significant? My whole body had been poisoned—how could anything have survived that? I refused to get riled up. I had my previously scheduled Mayo appointment within the month. I would bring it to my doctor's attention at that time. I could wait two weeks. I wouldn't even tell Tom. No sense in alarming anyone for no reason. I'd casually mention it to my doctor, and I knew he would reassure me and life would proceed without incident.

One of the girls from the dentist office I work in was able to go with me to Mayo for my checkup. Sandy was always up for an adventure. I really appreciated that about her. She was a lot of fun and we talked all the way to Mayo.

I went through all the testing, and the doctor said everything looked great. I decided now was the time, and I brought up the lump on the left side. The doctor felt it and said they needed to investigate it. Mind you, this was Friday before Memorial Day. It looked as if many people had already left for the long weekend. At 3 p.m. they did the biopsy, and at 6 p.m. my doctor came in and informed me the cells didn't look good. The full pathology couldn't be done until Tuesday. I knew. I just knew. I knew this was Dr. S's way of telling me it was back to the drawing board. My wall crumbled.

Sandy consoled and cried with me. She was left to fill the gap. I felt terrible that she was in that role, but I couldn't control my emotions. She had been instantly called into "breast friend" duty. You never know who you are going to pull into service when the storm comes.

Tom called while I was still at Mayo. I told him about the bad-looking cells, and that they were doing more extensive testing. I told him that I would explain when I got home. I said it didn't look good. He didn't ask any more questions. He didn't jump to the obvious conclusion, but he knew I was upset.

The ride home was not the flow of laughter and conversation that the drive to Mayo had been. Sandy and I were seven hours from home. It seemed endless. Even still, it wasn't long enough to figure out how to tell my family. The disbelief of it all was crushing. Sandy listened quietly as I rambled on about what this all would mean again. Mile after mile. How could I do this again? The thought of it all was incomprehensible. Cancer had changed my life once before and now I was facing it again. I knew what was ahead of me this time, and it wasn't comforting. Was I never to be free of this thing called cancer? Would I never stop hearing my possible death sentence read over and over? I remember telling Sandy, "I can't do this again." The anger started to boil up inside of me. I hesitated to be as angry as I really felt in front of Sandy. It wasn't her fault. She was an innocent bystander to my cancer saga. She was great. I couldn't have asked for a more supportive "breast friend." I was not so good.

I thanked Sandy when our drive finally came to an end and apologized for the predicament she had endured. She smiled sweetly and reassured me. I appreciated her kindness.

The second scene of telling my family of cancer's return played out a little differently than the first time. Saturday morning everyone was seated at the kitchen table. Tom announced the bad news to the family: Mom has a new tumor. We will be dealing with breast cancer again. This news hit us all differently this time. The kids crumbled into tears. They were fully aware of what this meant. Tom stated how we would fight this again and that we would *all* get through it. I heard his strong words and yet looked into my children's desperate and sad eyes. I hated cancer for doing this all over again. Normal life would be shoved back in the closet. I was once again the bearer of bad news and new schedules. Schedules that didn't revolve around being the mother and wife I wanted to be. My oldest daughter seemed heavy with the weight of this news. She was home from college for the summer, and this would change her role in the household. I didn't want that for her. I didn't want to rely on her. I knew she didn't want to have to be relied on. Tom was going into his second reelection. There was no other option.

I called Mayo Tuesday morning after the holiday. It was confirmed. It was definitely cancer. The following weekend, Tom and I decided to leave for an impromptu visit to Mackinac Island. He had a conference he was expected at, and Mayo confirmed that the time would have no impact on treatment. There was no need to rush. I knew what was waiting for me. We left our oldest in charge, and I headed off with Tom to try and wrap my brain around my situation. The drive started the process of my acceptance back into the world of cancer.

It's hard to believe, but we had a good time on this trip. Tom had several colleagues on the island for the Detroit Chamber Conference. Word had traveled fast about my cancer. We were notified by one of Tom's colleagues that they would be having a prayer meeting for me, and they wanted us to attend. We were both very touched by this kindness and made plans to be there. There was a group of twenty people in the room by the time we showed up. It was overwhelming to me that these complete strangers would take the time to pray for me. They all knew Tom, but not me. While they were praying, I could feel myself make the transition from anger about my condition to acceptance. I told myself the fight would be on again. I had done this before, and I could do it again. That group of quietly praying people allowed me to process what I would have to do

The Lord had truly prepared me through Nikki. I thought back to the dinner party and the conversation with her at the door. I was in awe that my sense that something was on the horizon had been confirmed. I had no idea at that time just what the significance of that conversation would be. Apparently, the Lord was already working, and I had been left to catch up. I knew He would be right there with me again. It was time to believe in my own words again. Why I had to endure this once more might never be answered clearly, but putting the Lord in charge was a given.

The Monday after we had returned home from the conference, Tom and I again headed out on the road. This time it wasn't to a lovely resort but to Mayo. The ease and comfort of the previous weekend had vanished, and conversation was difficult. I knew Tom was trying to be strong and wanted a way to fix this. Every other thought in our heads had been swept away, and both of us were focused on cancer again. Things that we normally would have talked about didn't seem very relevant or worthy of our time right now. Tom was in the "wait and see" mode, while I was in "let's get this over with" mode. I wanted to get right into whatever plan of action was necessary to get this out of my life once and for all. If they had been able to FedEx the solution, I would have plugged it into the car. Not very practical, but action would have been comforting.

We never talked about my dying. Oh, I thought about it, and I know Tom probably did as well. It was the chair in the room that no one would sit in. Obviously empty, but empty on purpose. I would have talked about it. Not because I wanted to talk about my death. Nobody wants to discuss their death, but talking about it was a way to process through it or at least ramble on until exhaustion and resignation ruled. But I believe for Tom, talking about it would have made it too real. He and I both knew the second time was a more serious event. We both knew stories of cancer rearing its ugly self again only to end badly. We weren't novices about what was ahead. I knew Tom's goal was to be uplifting, and I would let him fulfill that job while I coped with being the cause of all of this.

We arrived at Mayo, and my first consultation was about my new lump. My personal plan of action was to remove the lump and go through the chemo and come back for a full mastectomy at a later date. I didn't have time for all of this right now, and I didn't want to make any more time for cancer than necessary. I could minimize the family impact right now and schedule the big show at a later, more convenient date. The doctors talked about their plan of action. Tom did a lot more listening, while I ran through possible scenarios and thought about my calendar.

My doctor explained that the Tamoxifen obviously didn't do the job that they had expected. She was very concerned. Tom looked at me in disbelief as the questions flowed out of my mouth. I knew he thought I was dictating to them how they were going to handle me, instead of me listening to their strategy. I was focused on dealing with the relative simplicity of a lumpectomy, so I wouldn't have to disturb my eighteen-month-old reconstructed breast that I was very pleased with. I wasn't ready to face a double full mastectomy. I could tell what they were thinking, and I could live with a dent in my breast rather than no breasts at all. I'm sure a stranger would have looked at Tom and me as two people who had two totally separate conversation bubbles above our heads with nothing connecting the two.

The doctor sympathized with my feelings but insisted on a MRI before any other decisions. She needed to see if anything else was going on medically in my body. She explained that although my situation wasn't unique, it wasn't a common occurrence. I had remembered hearing that the first time you have cancer, they throw both barrels at you, so if it happens again, the concern level increases. Tom was comforted by the continual testing. I was irritated that they weren't cooperating with my timeline.

After the MRI, I found I not only had the tumor in my left breast, but that I had cancerous cells in my right breast. I knew instantly that there was no saving "the girls," even the fake one. Tom was all set to have them get every inch of contaminated flesh off immediately. I, on the other hand, was livid. Why hadn't they been screening me with MRIs all along, if this could detect all these cells? They informed me that: a) it's not the preferred screening method; b) insurance doesn't cover this consistently; and c) it is only when a problem presents itself that they use it as a diagnostic tool. I was seriously disappointed at this matter-of-fact strategy and furious that I had cancer taking up residence in me all this time, when it could have been spotted earlier. I knew this would mean full mastectomy, even though I wasn't exactly sure what that would all entail. How were they going to put "the girls" back together again? Maybe it wouldn't be an option. What were the options? What happens when you have cancer the second time? My mind was racing. I knew Tom had to be as stunned as I was. I knew he would be focused on curing me while I was focused on my potential deformity.

The plan was to return the following week to coordinate with surgeons so that reconstruction could proceed as quickly as possible. I had made it very clear that my reconstruction was my prime objective. I wasn't going to dilly dally again. I knew that the sooner I got those expanders in, the sooner I could resume my normal life, looking like my normal self. I caught Tom's look of disbelief as I asserted my demands. I knew he was completely dumbfounded by my focus, compared to his goal of getting me cancer free. In my mind there was no reason why we couldn't accomplish both goals at the same time.

I knew back home the whole family would think I was dead for sure this time. The whole treatment regimen would have to start again. In the back of my mind I figured maybe they could do a lumpectomy. That would save time! No, probably not. Why? Why was neither cancer diagnosed with mammograms? Boy was I ticked. My question list grew exponentially as I sat listening to the plan being laid out. I could feel my anger rising. My anger wasn't for the doctors; it was for the situation I found myself in again. I wasn't looking forward to the three days of testing and turmoil.

The testing finished up after a couple of days. I can't even remember all the tests they did. I would return the following Tuesday for my mastectomy surgery. It would be coordinated with the reconstruction surgeon, my trusted friend, Dr. T. So, I congratulated myself that I had successfully eliminated one surgery and sped the process in the direction I desired.

Tom and I went home. The weekend was a needed break. Decisions had been made. The fort would be secured, and I could mentally regroup for Tuesday. The kids were busy with their various jobs and activities. I knew they were holding back any demands and working to accommodate this newest round of life change.

A blessing presented itself to us during this weekend. A local flight group offered to shuttle Tom and me to Mayo for surgery and back home afterwards. The thought of being able to be back in my own bedroom quickly after the surgeons had taken their pound of flesh was a comforting thought for me. Tom and I gratefully accepted.

Tom and I flew out on Tuesday morning. It was a beautiful day. You would never have guessed that we were heading to Mayo and not off to some romantic location. It was exciting to climb into this little plane. I needed this distraction. Anything that kept my mind off what was ahead was greatly appreciated. I scanned the plane with all its instruments and little seats. Our pilot was Bob T. He is a dear friend of ours now, but at the time he was my plane angel. I'll call him that instead of a "breast friend," considering he's a guy. He was my quick ticket to home. Bob and Tom sat in the front while I climbed in the back. Soon I settled in back with the rest of the necessary plane decor, while the boys bonded over politics and flight in the front. Their endless conversation gave me the opportunity to stare out the window at the beauty I was flying above. I focused on all the little houses and wondered if any were full of the drama that was playing out in my life. They looked so peaceful surrounded by happy fields of green and undisturbed forests. Soon the landscape changed to a busyness of suburbia and then to full-out city. We were ready to land. *Here we go,* I thought. Tom and I thanked our plane angel and grabbed a taxi to Mayo.

Once Tom and I were at Mayo, we got our hotel room. We had one more night before the surgery. We settled into our room, and my mind began to race. Waves of emotion washed over me. I felt as if I were in a hurricane. Tom assured me of his love and that he didn't care about the physical aspect. I questioned and pushed trying to catch any sign that he would be disappointed or that this was overwhelming or that somehow he had been cheated. Instead, his words reassured me, and he was crystal clear … nothing could change his heart.

Chapter Thirty-Two

SURGERY AGAIN

$\mathscr{S}$oon the alarm was going off, and we had to head to the hospital to check in. The busyness of this kept us moving forward. I couldn't think of anything but the next thing I had to do. But soon, there I was again, laying in pre-op. Another pre-op. I'd been in this position before. Unfortunately, I knew how this went. Tom couldn't be with me now. There I lay all by myself. Tears streamed down my face. I felt like that lamb stuck in the thicket with a wolf staring at me. The wolf was coming, and I knew he would get me. I knew I would survive the attack, but part of me would be missing. My tears were interrupted by the occasional visit of my surgeons. They asked their polite questions and tried to comfort me in the two minutes they had to spare, but it wasn't enough. How could it be? So they did the next best thing and handed me the box of Kleenex. I couldn't control the rapid-fire thoughts and images that were racing through my brain. It was a relief when they placed the IV and my lids began to close. Time stopped for me.

Light filtered through my lids as I began to awake. Slowly, my mind was bringing me back to reality. The first sensation

I had was the feeling that an elephant was sitting on my chest. There didn't seem to be a great deal of pain, but there was a lot of pressure. I could feel the emotion begin to well up inside of me as the tears started again. Thoughts were racing through my brain faster than I could deal with them. What had happened while I was in surgery? Had they found more cancer? Was the cancer in my lymph nodes? Were they able to place the expanders? Could I make it through this process again? What would I see when the bandages came off this time? Each question came and went without an answer. I could guess, but nothing was clear yet. It was all still up for grabs at this point.

Then I remembered … the doctor had warned me that breast surgery was particularly hard on the emotions and that I should expect it to be disruptive to my train of thought. He had also said that I probably wouldn't feel like myself and that mood swings could be dramatic. It was turning out to be true. I felt it taking place as I lay there. One after another, the emotions rolled over me. There were so many that I lay there in disbelief. Thank goodness he had warned me, or I would have been shocked by the extremes. All of it was punctuated by my tears.

Soon, Tom was with me. He immediately began to reassure me, and I knew his goal was to be supportive. He searched for the right words to console me. Again, I heard the words I needed to hear from him. "I love you and nothing could ever change that." He assured me he wasn't in love with my breasts. He told me how brave I was and how proud he was that I had come this far so well. His words began to soothe my troubled mind, and I felt my hands slowly unclench. I knew that it was me who would have the more difficult time accepting the massive change to my body. I couldn't go backwards. It was done. We both were getting good at accepting, moving forward, and focusing on being positive. We knew the Lord was in control. This plan was the winner over and over again.

Tom and I were both anxious to speak to the doctors, and soon there was a whole entourage of doctors filling my room. This couldn't be good. Why were there so many? I'm sure there were other sick people who needed attending to. My breast surgeon led the way and began to introduce his colleagues and the several interns to Tom and me. We both smiled tentatively at the group. I wondered if the group was for me or for the protection for the doctor after he informed me of the findings of surgery. I suppose people handled these things in all different manners. Maybe doctors felt more comfortable if they had company during a pronouncement on someone's life. We were going to find out.

The doctor began to speak. He announced that the cancer had not spread to my lymph nodes, and no cancer was in the surrounding tissues. He appeared to be very pleased with his speech. I know Tom and I were very pleased. Then, Dr. T, my reconstruction surgeon, began to happily tell me that he had been able to place the expanders during my surgery. He said that I was very fortunate because this is rarely done at the time of a complete mastectomy. With a gleam in his eye he said, "Mrs. Casperson, I don't know how many times I'm going to have to reconstruct you; you are special." At that moment, I really did feel special and incredibly cared for. It was like I was the only one in the hospital, and I think Dr. T was as pleased with himself as he was with my surgery.

As soon as the good news express was over, the interns took over. They began to discuss the case among themselves and ask questions. There were a lot of questions. I didn't mind all the activity. Having all of them there quickly lightened the mood now that the silence and seriousness had been broken. Soon they were all leaving, tossing cheery and positive wishes my way. What a great group of doctors these interns would be someday. They were the best of the best doctors anywhere. I felt blessed to be in their caring hands. The room had emptied, and it was back to Tom and me alone again.

A young couple found their way to my room. They peeked in and asked if they could visit with us. Tom eagerly invited them in. This woman explained that she had just come through the same surgery. She described her own battle with cancer and how she felt. It could have been me standing there, because the facts were so similar. After she finished her story, we continued to share small talk, and our men did the same. We all talked eagerly as if we had known each other forever, and this was a great help to Tom and me. We realized we weren't all alone in this predicament. This appeared to be yet another divine appointment in our tiny hospital room and more people to add to my list of "breast friends." I don't remember their names, but I know that they deserve the credit for helping Tom and me to take our first step to healing. So, wherever they are ... thank you. God is so good!

The next day, we headed for home. Once again I left the hospital with the familiar drain tubes hanging out my sides. I was wrapped tighter than a sausage, which was a good thing. I didn't want to see the scalpel's work just yet. Again, we were blessed to be able to take the quick flight home. When we arrived at the airport, the plane was waiting for us. I was so thankful to be able to avoid the long car ride that it normally would have taken from Mayo back to our small town.

Getting into the plane was my only challenge. The pilot looked at me reassuringly and at Tom for guidance. Tom, on the other hand, looked like he was measuring how to place me into the plane. I appreciated his tenderness, and I don't think he could have been any gentler. It was as if all of my 206 bones had been broken and it was up to him to carefully organize them into the plane. Our pilot was sympathetic yet stoic. He left the organizing to Tom. I couldn't have felt any safer or loved. Once the final positioning was done, we began our flight. It was over before I knew it, and we arrived at our local airport.

I hadn't phoned the kids since the surgery. I just wanted to see them once I was home. I had, however, notified my mother. She would meet our plane. I knew she would want to hear as soon as possible what the plans for me would be. I know, as a mom, standing by and waiting for news about your child is unbearable. I don't think that feeling ever changes, no matter how old your children get to be. I knew I had put my mom through too many days of worrying already.

Delicately, Tom unloaded his precious cargo … me. I spotted my mother's face. I could see the relief written on it, and I was glad she was there. Tom and I said our thank-you to the pilot, and off we all headed to the kids who were waiting. It was a great homecoming. There were signs and banners everywhere. There were plants and flowers of every kind. Love and cheers of welcome filled the air. Even more noticeable was the state of the house. The kids had cleaned everything. Their aim was to please and comfort, and they had succeeded. Nothing says I love you to me like the smell of clean and shining stainless. It was great to be home. Now, I don't recommend cancer to get this kind of effort out of kids, but I was pleased. Obviously, years of training had actually sunk in. Hooray!

Tom and I spent a small amount of time processing through the past days' events. The kids had questions. Mostly, they wanted to know if I would be all right again? We reassured them it would be another lengthy process; but that it looked good and that I had done it before and could do it again. I really believed that. I didn't like that it was all starting again, but I was home … and that was positive. I was ushered to my bed, and there I settled in.

Each day I improved in both strength and in spirit. Everyone worked very hard to make my recuperation peaceful. Even the dog was careful. They always seem to know when something is up, and she was no exception.

The sausage wrap came off after two days. The doctor had given me instructions on when and how to do this. My first look at myself was not what I had expected. They had told me they had been able to put the expanders in during the surgery. What would that look like? Well ... it looked like two gentle rises in a pretty flat landscape. Now, you might be thinking, Awww, that's disappointing. No, no, no, I was okay with it. There was no concave look, and that was a big improvement from the first time I had been down this road. Yeah it was 34 AAAA, but at least a measurement could be taken. *This is very good,* I thought to myself.

Even though I knew breasts were severely overrated compared to my life, I was glad to see a step towards normalcy! I could recognize the progress that had already been made towards reconstruction. This helped to calm my worries of the unknown and the anticipation of how this was all going to work. I could deal with this. No, I wasn't happy with the results yet, but I wasn't falling to pieces, and I knew I was already ten steps ahead of the game with the expanders in place. The new "me" was emerging in a small but positive way. Dr. T may never have known at the time how this helped me take a giant leap forward in the acceptance of the new me and the calming of my fears. Having been through this process before, I knew in my heart how huge this was to my recovery.

My life proceeded calmly, and I continued to build up my strength. Tom and I returned to Mayo two weeks later to discuss further treatment and to check my progress. Well, turned out it wasn't all roses and champagne corks. The cancerous tumor they had removed was more than 2 mm in size. This meant that the oncologist was recommending chemo again. I hoped my face didn't look as stunned and disappointed as Tom's, but I'm sure it must have. The doctors informed us that my type of breast cancer was again estrogen positive. This cancer was just like the first cancer had been. The doctors voiced their concerns about future tumors and the role that estrogen could play in growing them. They explained how they recommended a full hysterectomy when this was the case. They said this was needed to eliminate estrogen, the culprit in my own body.

Really? I thought to myself. *Did I just hear them tell me that I needed a full hysterectomy?* I could once again feel the tears building. Here was another blow to my womanhood, at least what little was left of it. There would officially be nothing left to confirm my being feminine. I couldn't believe that this was happening again. How many more times would I have to hear a stranger tell me what parts of my body they needed to remove for my own good?

The doctors quickly switched to the "silver lining" in all of this. They announced there was no spread of cancer and no lymph nodes were involved. They stressed that this was very good news, and that the worry of future cancer was now on hold. Their voices trailed off as I remembered hearing these same words six years earlier. I had thought then that I was done with cancer. I know the look on my face was less than confident, and that if I had a "yippee" to give, it wouldn't be a very excited one. I knew what this all meant for my life. It meant I was once again in the trenches fighting cancer. Except this time, my breasts were already gone.

Strangely enough, that was a comfort. At first it didn't seem that way, but quickly I began to realize that my radical decision had eliminated the possibility of cancer ever hiding out in breast tissue again. It was the one decision I had been able to make for myself, and I was glad I had chosen that option. The rest of the decisions about my body would be made by my team of doctors.

There would be no contemplating options. Oh, sure they would be polite and include me, but they knew what needed to be done to give me the best possible odds at survival. I had no choice but to accept my marching orders.

My hysterectomy would be done at Mayo. I decided to have it done there for my own peace of mind. I would follow up with my local doctor at home for the chemo treatments. There would be no radiation this time. They informed me that there was nothing left to radiate. Well, that was a bright spot.

After pondering all the new treatment plans, I started thinking about all the havoc estrogen could be having in the rest of my body. Fresh off a surgery, I couldn't shake the idea that cancer could be lurking somewhere else. What about ovarian, or uterine, or any other sneaky cancer roaming around? They recommended twelve weeks of chemo. I wanted to have the hysterectomy first and then the rounds of chemo. June was the mastectomy, July was my hysterectomy, first of August chemo began. What a fun summer. Once again, I would be heading into the holidays after chemo. There was no radiation required because there wasn't anything to radiate. Lucky me. It was like déjà vu; I had almost the exact same timeline as the first round of cancer. Once again, I figured the sooner I got started, the sooner I'd be done.

Because it was 2006, my husband was again running for public office. I didn't want to pull him away from the campaign for another one of my surgeries. He gladly would have taken me for the hysterectomy, but my sister Linda offered to come home and take me. She said she would be glad to do it. That would allow Linda and me to have our own road trip. It would give us time to visit. Share like only sisters can share. I knew I could tell Linda anything, and I knew she would listen and give me the comfort I needed. All the details were shored up, and before too long we were on our way.

Linda and I arrived the day before the surgery. Modern hysterectomy surgery requires only one night of hospital stay. It was an open-and-shut case. There were no surprises, and they informed me in post op that there was no cancer anywhere. No cancer! Hooray … no cancer anywhere! My whole body began to unwind with the news. One more hurdle was done. The news couldn't have been any better. Linda had listened as intently as I did. Her relief was as evident as mine, and she responded to my every need. I already knew she was a special sister, but our trip confirmed that she wasn't just my beloved sister but a "breast friend."

The next day Linda and I headed home. Everything had gone as planned. It was wonderful to get home. Once again, the house had been readied with flowers and cards. How many times could people be so kind? Everywhere I looked were plants and cards from loved ones and well-wishers. My kids had once again put on their most loving smiles.

I took the minimum of three weeks off of work. Now, no letters from all you gals who've had hysterectomies because I know everybody's recovery time is different. For me, I needed my life to begin again as quickly as possible. You take as long as you need in this process. I needed to fill my days with life-giving activity. I was tired but I needed to be around others and hear and see the basic rhythm of everyday life. I was anxious to start chemo again and finish the last leg of my treatment. The sooner I got going, the sooner it would be behind me.

Chemo was another twelve weeks marked on my calendar. I would have one treatment every Friday. I chose to have this administered at my local hospital. Thank you to the special "breast friends" who took up their post each Friday with me during treatment. You know who you are, and your quiet strength and presence held me together. Thank you.

I was pretty down all summer. It wasn't due to lack of support. Chemo just takes its toll. I still worked, but my friends frequently came in and saved the day. They arrived with dinner, cleaning crews, and plenty of plants. Even with all the help I received, my role as mom still took a hit. When my oldest daughter came home from college, she stepped up to the plate and took charge. Her can-do attitude prevailed, and she filled in for me in a lot of ways. I know it wasn't easy for her to be in that role, but she did it. It also helped that the other kids were older this time around. They knew more than the first time I had cancer and were able to make some of the adjustments needed. They were more self-sufficient and worked hard to ease the strain of each situation. Even though they were better, I didn't like that they had to deal with a sick mother. This is one of the things that you can't control. Cancer once again forces you to rely on others, and I was no different.

Chapter Thirty-Three

CHEMO AND THE ELECTION

*C*hemo was actually pretty uneventful. I know it's hard to believe that I would describe chemo as uneventful, but I had been able to keep my schedule fairly normal until the very end. I took extra rest when I needed it, and friends had continued to rally to my aid.

I had successfully gotten to my eleventh treatment. That meant I only had one left. That treatment came the Friday before Tom's third Election Day. As a family, we were feeling very positive that Tom would be successful. I went through the weekend feeling fine, and soon it was election night. We were gathered with all of Tom's supporters at the election-night party where we learned that Tom had won. I was very happy for Tom and relieved it was over. Elections are an exhausting process in themselves. I excused myself early from the election party because I wasn't feeling 100 percent. Not that I had a clear picture of what 100 percent was, but I wasn't feeling good and I didn't think anyone would mind me leaving after the results were known. I told Tom I was heading home and reassured him that I was just tired.

I remember crawling into bed thinking something was wrong. I knew chemo kills your ability to fight off even the smallest of intruders, so I thought maybe it was the flu. I felt chilled but pushed those thoughts out of my head and focused on sleep. I didn't hear Tom come home that night, but I was awakened at 4 a.m. to my body trembling uncontrollably. I grabbed the thermometer and took my temperature: 105. I could tell by the look on Tom's face that he thought I was checking out. I must have looked as bad as I felt. I could feel the panic in him, and it was threatening to overtake me. I knew this wasn't good. Tom rushed me to the emergency room where we asked that they notify my oncologist.

They quickly admitted me and started the testing. They soon surmised that I had a blood infection from the port that had been installed to ease the administration of the chemo. Immediately, I was infused with antibiotics. I was in the hospital for several days. Again, I was flat on my back in a hospital. No hair, no strength, the new chemo girl on the block. Doctors and nurses were once again racing around me searching for answers. I was tired of being in the middle of this medical typhoon. Ultimately, they were able to find the right antibiotic to fight the infection, and after it was under control, my oncologist conceded the last treatment of chemo. Eleven treatments would have to do. They removed the port and called it "good." That was fine with me. I'd take my chances with eleven instead of twelve. As soon as I was physically able, I was getting my show out of another hospital. I was seriously tired of hospitals.

So, to recap: Thanksgiving was here again, then Christmas. Two thousand and six was one year I was looking to put to rest. May was the diagnosis of my second round of breast cancer. June was a complete mastectomy. July was a complete hysterectomy, followed by eleven weeks of chemo. November was the election, followed by red-alert blood infection. December, I was glad to be alive … priceless. Come on 2007.

Chapter Thirty-Four

RECONSTRUCTION

$\mathcal{B}$ecause of the surgery and chemo, the filling of the expanders had been on hold. Now that surgery and chemo were in the rearview mirror, it was time to resume the reconstruction process. Surprise, surprise: another breast friend put on her cape and came to my aid. Sharon would come to my home every two weeks to fill the expanders. She had more of a job than the first time I had this done, since there were two sides to fill. It was a more elaborate process, and she knew it would take about six months to get the expanders where they needed to be. This process was long and painful. I so appreciated her time and energy. We often laughed about the predicament we found ourselves in. Not everyone gets the unique experience of having a friend help them stretch their muscles for the placement of future breasts. Cancer had forced me into intimate situations that formed bonds out of my personal weakness. Funny thing is that those bonds are precious for that very reason. You are special, Sharon.

Now, you'd hardly think that all this fuss over fake breasts would be worth it, but I wanted to look normal again. I could be patient with this process, and I felt that I had earned the right to try to look okay again. Dr. T had assured me that if I was patient, I would be happy with the end results. I trusted Dr. T, so I followed his instructions to the letter and began the process of reconstruction again.

Chapter Thirty-Five

CHICAGO

*I*t was January again, and although I was happy about my reconstruction, I fell into that sluggish, unmotivated state that is post chemo. The all-too-familiar winter blues set in, and the thought of exercise or returning to the YMCA to give me motivation sounded ridiculous and repetitive. Everything sounded ridiculous and repetitive. Even though my previous experience had been so uplifting, I couldn't bring myself to do it all again. I stumbled through February and into March.

April would bring a new challenge. Remember Jan from earlier in my story? She became the newest divine appointment in my life, another "breast friend" sent to guide me into another new phase of recovery. I didn't recognize it at the time, but I figure the Lord knew I would need a fresh approach and He provided.

Jan's carefully devised plan was to approach me about a cancer walk, which she did. I flatly told her "no" at first. I had already been down the victorious marathon road, and the inspiration to repeat an exhausting goal just wasn't there for me. My previous marathon had been an incredible experience, and I was grateful for it, but I couldn't muster the enthusiasm to do anything that resembled it again. I didn't think it was possible to recapture the specialness of it all.

Jan kept up her subtle attack and stuck to the idea that this walk would be a great way to jump-start my energy and speed me back into normalcy. When Jan saw that I wasn't going for the challenge, she would switch gears and we would talk about our lives and its demands. She had three children, and we shared our mothering stories. She was very good at not pushing her marathon agenda. Jan convinced me that we could just walk for the health of it, with no expectations on her part. She wanted a partner to walk with to prepare herself, and I agreed.

We set a date and went for our first walk. We walked for two miles. The time had sped by, and I was shocked that I was able to go for two miles. It turned out I really wasn't as pathetic as I had led myself to believe. This second cancer hadn't taken me all the way down physically like I was giving it credit for.

We still walked with no commitment from me towards any goal, and Jan seemed satisfied with that. They were casual walks with pleasant conversation. We did this for a month before she brought up the cancer walk again. She later told me that through our conversations, she had picked up that I needed a reason to step outside my door again. She told me that it was a purpose that had been placed on her heart. We had a shared faith, and we marveled at the direction our relationship had taken. Jan informed me how she believed that she and her husband had been relocated so that she could accomplish this mission. I couldn't comprehend being someone's mission.

How I had been given such a gift still mystifies me, but at the time I didn't have any idea of the big picture that was being painted. When Jan asked again, I said yes. The goal seemed more appealing than when we had first discussed it. I now looked at it as a way to push me over the hurdle of sickness again and back to health. Jan had been successful in her gentle approach. Besides, this was a walk not a run, I told myself.

We had two months to train for the Chicago Avon Walk. This would be a two day, forty-mile walk. Training took more time than energy. It was walking for hours on end. I can't even tell you the miles we logged and the things we passed. To this day, we both still have several cows that we had passed on our walks that we endearingly named. I'm sure those cows had no idea the motivation for our frequent visits through their territory. As a matter of fact, I'm sure they failed to notice us after the first few times.

Conversation was never lacking for Jan and me. That's a true testament to a woman's ability to relate. Personally, being a woman provides so much material, it's hard to find a reason to be quiet. People asked how we could walk for so long. Honestly, it wasn't that hard at all—time consuming, but not hard. I felt like I was spending time with someone who was helping to sew my spirit back together. Walking mile after mile with a person reveals who they are and what they believe. The long distances were a challenge physically, but I was left with a good "ache." I was beginning to feel my energy and vitality return.

The walk required that we raise $1800 per participant for cancer research. We put out the call for donations. Collectively, we were able to raise over $13,000 for the cause. We were astonished. Friends and family were generous beyond belief, and I was amazed at how quickly the funds accumulated. I felt so honored to be the bearer of such an offering.

But as usual, some people questioned my ability after what I had been through. They had trouble understanding why I would take on such a monumental task. I was alive … wasn't that good enough for me? I asked myself, Why was I doing this? Well, once again, I can only say that somehow I needed this. The Lord had placed it before me, and I felt as if my steps were ordered. Jan felt the same. I reaffirmed to myself that once again I needed to walk cancer out of my life in a powerful way and hoped that I would be able to walk hope into others that I knew would be there ready to be new "breast friends". As survivors, we were in this fight for our lives and our very souls. So, I shrugged off the negativity the same way I had needed to shrug off death and fear and separation in order to really live.

I found it ironic that I was in Chicago again. It was May 2007. This was just one year past the start of my second cancer journey. This was a different event, but once again I was surrounded by thousands of potential "breast friends." There were over 4,500 walkers registered for this event. Some were survivors, some were in the midst of the battle, and some walked in memory of loved ones lost. I felt like there was nowhere else on earth that Jan and I needed to be than right where we were. I had total peace that we could do this.

The walk required us to be on our feet for 26.3 miles the first day. This was no easy task even after all our training. It would be two days of enormous effort.

By the second day, we were feeling the strain, and it showed in the walkers all around us. Not everyone was able or prepared for the grueling pace of this endeavor. We saw the people filling the aid stations with various physical complaints, but we continued on our path with our eyes focused. Jan and I were thankful to be able to complete the walk. Our preparation and God's grace had allowed us to claim the finish line in victory. We weren't first and we weren't last, but we had finished, and that was all that mattered to us. It was exhilarating. Here I was, again able to walk cancer out of my life. God's abundant mercy had once again blessed me with a new inner and outer strength to deal with whatever life had to offer. Thank you, Jan, for being a true conduit for a greater plan than I could have ever imagined.

Chapter Thirty-Six

LOOKING BACK

*N*ormal life returned almost as fast as it had disappeared, and two years have passed more quickly than I could imagine. Looking back, I can evaluate things more clearly than when I was in the midst of cancer. Mistake number one: thinking like a girl. Admit it. Everyone has an idea of her "pretty." Not model pretty, because models don't even think they're pretty, but the "hey, I look good in this, and there's no apparent reason why others shouldn't agree with that" kind of pretty. Sure, everything is subject to opinion, but given the girl standards, I'm passable. My husband must've seen something that was agreeable to him. Like most women, that's important to me too. I mean, what if I started cutting things off of my body? This would be changing the package he fell in love with. Now, don't get me wrong. The package had changed over the years. I did have four children, and a life. All the pieces were still there and functioning. Are you getting the mistake being made here? My husband wasn't putting any expectations on me. My husband was dealing with my potential death. He didn't care if I had one breast, two breasts, or three. I wasn't giving him enough credit. It was me that was still learning what was important, and my hesitations were my problem and not my husband's or my family's.

Mistake number two: time management. How long would recovery take? Was there a way to streamline this process? Was there an efficient way to manage cancer and how it was going to interrupt my schedule? I didn't want to have too much distraction for my family. Yeah it was cancer, but I thought I could dig deep and power through. You might be thinking that same thing right now. Good. It means you're a fighter. However, it also means you're someone who could neglect yourself. Remember, cancer won't let you neglect yourself. It yells, "stop, you better pay attention to me. I'm waging a physical war on you, and you better respond properly or you're going to regret it." I wasn't so good at heeding that message at first. But, you need to hang on to your fighting because you're going to need it to get going again.

Mistake number three: don't underestimate yourself or others. You will surprise yourself, and others will surprise you. Sometimes it will be negative, but most times it will be positive. Always resort to love. It truly does conquer all, and you'll never regret showing it.

Finally, the most often made mistake: perfection. Guess what? I made mistakes, and I still do. I realized that cancer can't be managed perfectly. It changes you. You let it for your own good. Bending is always preferable to breaking. Sometimes you can control the impact, and sometimes you can't. Realize that it's a fluid process. Cut yourself some slack.

Chapter Thirty-Seven

PRESENT DAY

I am happy, healthy, and I have two wonderful breasts that fill up my bra. I know you can't believe I'm going to say this, but cancer left me with better hair and two perky, newly reconstructed breasts. A friend gave me a shirt, and on occasion, I wear it with a grin and a sense of how precious life is. It says, "Of course these are fake ... my real ones tried to kill me!" But on the serious side, I hope I continue to wear my suit of thankfulness as openly as I did on the day of my oldest daughter's wedding. I have three more children and a husband that I look forward to marking all life's milestones with. This book has allowed me to finally express the things I've learned through cancer: how God's promptings have blessed me, and how thankfulness is a learned choice. I choose thankfulness. Every day is a treasure. Sometimes it's gold bullion and other days it's wrapped chocolate.

Cancer is always at the back of my brain. It doesn't control my life, but it will never leave me. Just like all of those horrific experiences that shape us, we are never completely free, but hopefully we are better. We are all called to be better. If I have helped to walk anyone through this experience with comfort or laughter and a few honest tears, I am grateful for that opportunity.

I'm not famous, but cancer is. Through cancer I have been blessed by many mentors, family, and friends. There is life after cancer. In some ways life is better. Better in that I couldn't have walked this journey without my faith. Faith in Jesus Christ who bore far more that I ever could even imagine. I am reminded often of the Scripture in Matthew 7:24-27, where I believe it teaches us to build our house on the rock and not sand, so that when the rains come and the winds blow, the house will not fall. So by building a firm foundation in Christ and trusting Him, we are equipped to handle the "storms" and heavy downpours in our lives without being swept away. We are left standing battered and bruised, but standing, hopeful for the future. We all have our battles and disappointments in life. None of us have been promised an easy life. We are called by Christ to accept, not understand. So, I hope this story will propel you in your walk through whatever it is you are facing and into a relationship with Jesus, because it truly is the only sure thing available to us humans.

What did I learn through this journey? First and foremost you need to be your own best advocate. No one will ask that extra question for you or be responsible for the level of education and knowledge needed about your own disease. Educating yourself is the greatest gift you can give yourself. It will help you to move forward and make better choices. It will help you evaluate your habits, both good and bad. It also provides you with qualifications to help mentor others. Today, I make better choices concerning my health and have worked to instill these values in my family. There have been changes in cancer treatment since my diagnosis and surgeries. There is more MRI use. I am grateful for that improvement in the spotting of and treatment of breast cancer.

The more quickly the problem is detected, the greater chance there is for a good outcome. Early detection is crucial. But mostly, like anything difficult in life, it is always in God's hands.

Finally, "breast friends" were provided all along the way to guide and shape my experience with cancer, but more importantly, with life. They lifted me when I couldn't lift myself and surrounded my family with love. I believe I am a wiser, more compassionate person due to the "breast friends" who ministered in my life. They taught me how to really care and provided a powerful example of how I can serve others. My faith has not been dimmed. It has become a beacon of rest and hope for me. I know where I need to go and how to get there when the waves start crashing and the fear starts rising. Is this difference because of cancer? Well, cancer was the catalyst for all this self-examination and others' outreach to me, but as I said before, I believe it's more. More about a teaching journey that now allows me to minister to others who are in the midst of their own personal storm. I have come to realize that if it is a storm like cancer that allowed me to be molded into a more humble and useful servant, then so be it. I have accepted my assignment and am *thankful* to have come through it.

A wise woman recently said to me, "The question is not why, the question should be, Lord what do you want me to do with this?"

ACKNOWLEDGMENTS

To my family:

My husband, Tom … Thank you for your unconditional love. You are my best friend, my rock, the love of my life.

My children, Ashley, Tommy, Hillary, and Dane … You are all so strong and often my voice of reason. You are each an example of God's blessing and mercy in my life, and I love you all more than life itself. I am thankful to be here to witness God's working in your lives.

My parents and siblings …Thank you for being a place of shelter and comfort. There's no better place than the arms of your mom—thanks.

To the Breast Friends in my life who deserve heartfelt acknowledgment:

Diane D. … You are my encourager, my mentor, and much more than a friend. Thank you.

Phyllis S. … You are my prayer warrior, an uplifting scriptural counselor, and a treasure. Thank you.

Kay Z. ... You taught me the meaning of "God knows" and helped me laugh through adversity. Thank you.

Connie C. ... Thank you for your hugs, your prayers, and your commitment to our friendship.

Sandi W. ... A dental patient turned mentor, turned friend. Thank you for your help and advice.

Jan M. ... A divine appointment that I am forever grateful for, and my forever friend. Thank you.

Laura S. ... The voice in my heart that points me to the "joy of the Lord [who] is our strength." I know she looks down on my survival with great pleasure. I miss her.

Marilyn E. ... My phone partner who is able to see far beyond her eyes' physical limitations. Thank you.

Charlene C. ... A coworker who soon became a time-honored friend. Thank you for always being there.

Debbie K. ... Another divine appointment designed to help nurse me back to health. Your physical strength was a catalyst for my own quest for strength and well-being. You are an amazing and true friend. Thank you.

Jean R. ... The bond we have is more than skin deep. There are no words that could capture my gratitude and the love I hold in my heart for you and your husband. Thank you.

Sharon Y. ... You are an example of unselfish love. Thank you.

Dr. Don ... Your kindness and understanding obviously knows no limit! Thanks, Boss.

Cyndi W. ... Funny what fate had in store for us. Not only have I gained an amazing "outlaw," but an amazing friend, without whose help this book would never have been possible.

To the doctors and nurses at Mayo Clinic ... You have the unique ability among the thousands of patients you see to make each one feel as if they are the only one. Without your compassion and dedication, my hope for success would have been greatly diminished. I send a special shout-out to Phyllis and Dr. T ... you are the best. Thank you.

Finally, there are many more people that I could have listed, and you know who you are. Every card, every gift, every act of kindness, every call, and mostly every prayer I am eternally grateful for. Thank you.

DIANE'S PERSONAL TESTIMONY:

My growing-up years had been happy years. I was very fortunate to have stable, loving parents and good friends. I had little difficulty fitting in. Yet, on the inside, I had a longing, an empty feeling that something was missing. Activities and the busyness of life can dull this for a while, but the hole remains.

Solomon, in the book of Ecclesiastes defines this void for us. He said, "God has put eternal life into the heart of every man" (3:11). The eternal life Solomon spoke of is played out in real-life question form. These questions are asked of everyone and always come in a group of three. These questions came to me.

My search started after I was married and Tom and I were thinking about having children. My husband and I were raised in different churches, and I wondered how we were we going to deal with this as a couple. What was important to us? We weren't involved in church functions but faithfully attended on Sundays for the most part. This was when the first question came from nowhere and began to bother me: "Who am I?" It puzzled me that I couldn't say who I really was. I didn't have time to dwell on the first question when the second followed: "What am I doing here?" This question was even deeper than the first. Finally, the third slammed into my thinking: "Where am I going?" I knew if I could find these answers, I would fill that hole I had been carrying around but that could no longer be ignored I now know these questions are from God. They are His way of ensuring that everyone would have a chance to know Him. Not just know of Him, but know Him in a personal way.

My intent is not to argue theology, but to share with you the moment that I believe changed my life forever. If you read the statistics, 80 percent of the U.S. population call themselves Christian. If you ask them why they are Christian, they will say they believe in God. I too fit this exact category. However, my beliefs were about to be challenged, and this would require me to get a lot more specific. A relative asked me, "Diane, when you die do you know where you will spend eternity?" I said, "I hope, I think heaven." And it was at that exact moment that life began to change for me and for Tom. Those next moments with my relative were to include plenty of Scripture, some of which I had never heard before. One of the Scripture verses was, "If you possess the Son, you possess life. If you do not possess the Son, you do not possess life. These things I have written unto you that you may know you have eternal life." (1 John 5:11-13) Wow, if that is true than how could I possess the Son ... because I sure want to know I have eternal life? Once again my relative pointed out with Scripture how this was possible. "Whoever calls on the name of the Lord will be saved" (Romans 10:1-3). The words came off the page as if they were written especially for me. The next Scripture I learned was in the same chapter in the book of Romans, and it said something everyone must know and believe. To me these words unfold right from the throne of God: "If you confess with your mouth that Jesus Christ is Lord and believe in your heart that God raised Him from the dead, you will be saved" (Romans 10:9-10). The simplicity of these directions by God took me by surprise. I could feel Him tugging at that emptiness in my heart. This was the way to fill that void. God was calling my name, and He is calling yours as well, if you don't know Him. On that day, in that moment, I prayed with my husband and asked Jesus to come into my heart, forgive me of my sin, and take over my entire life. In return, I promised Him I would do my best to serve Him every day of my life. I know that I will never be perfect in this endeavor, and that I will and have made plenty of mistakes since that moment. I now know that Christ doesn't call us to be perfect, because we are all sinners in need of a Savior.

As you have already read, my battle with cancer was certainly the single most difficult challenge of my life. Yet, I fully understand that God was not taken by surprise with my affliction. Rather, He knew that I would learn what most people have not. The most important thing in life is to love the Lord with all your heart. In return, I have found that He loves me more than I could possibly imagine.

You have heard people say, "There are many roads that lead to heaven." Don't believe that. There is only one way to eternal life, and Jesus tells us this, "I am the way, the truth and the life. No one comes to the Father but by me" (John 14:6). "For it is by grace you have been saved, through faith—and this not from yourselves, it is the gift of God—not by works, so that no one can boast. For we are God's handiwork, created in Christ Jesus to do good works, which God prepared in advance for us to do" (Ephesians 2:8-10). I realized that I couldn't earn my salvation, buy it, obtain it, or even live hoping for it by doing all the "right" things. It is a gift that I accepted.

I pray your three questions penetrate your heart, and you answer the most important of all as though you were standing before God. "Are you living for the Lord? If not, why not?" After all, there are no guarantees in life. However, this guarantee is absolute. If you make Jesus Christ the Lord of your life, you will never be the same, and He promises you a home forever with Him in heaven.

I hope that you will consider this a good work which God worked through me to offer to you.

God bless,
Diane

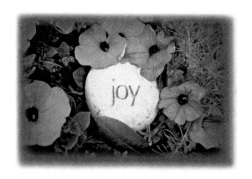

Reclaiming Your Joy

Can you find
Joy again on the
Path you now walk?
Do you know God's
Hand is sure as ever,
His grip not loosened
As you regain your balance

As you go down this path
Not able to see around
The next corner, He will
Nudge you forward,
To find joy waiting for
You, more wonderful
Because you thought it gone.

By Dean Schoen, Poems From the Crucible, 52 for You

Comments or questions to the author
or purchase of additional copies can be directed to
newbreastfriends@gmail.com

Additional copies of
New Breast Friends
Surviving Cancer...Twice
can be found at Barnes and Noble, Amazon.com
and all major bookstores

CPSIA information can be obtained at www.ICGtesting.com
Printed in the USA
BVOW071128290911

272350BV00001BA/4/P